T0130809

Management of the Charcot Foot and Ankle

Editor

BYRON HUTCHINSON

CLINICS IN PODIATRIC MEDICINE AND SURGERY

www.podiatric.theclinics.com

Consulting Editor
THOMAS J. CHANG

October 2022 • Volume 39 • Number 4

ELSEVIER

1600 John F. Kennedy Boulevard • Suite 1800 • Philadelphia, Pennsylvania, 19103-2899

http://www.theclinics.com

CLINICS IN PODIATRIC MEDICINE AND SURGERY Volume 39, Number 4
October 2022 ISSN 0891-8422, ISBN-13: 978-0-323-98659-5

Editor: Megan Ashdown
Developmental Editor: Diana Grace Ang

Clinics in Podiatric Medicine and Surgery (ISSN 0891-8422) is published quarterly by Elsevier Inc., 360 Park Avenue South, New York, NY 10010-1710. Months of issue are January, April, July, and October. Business and Editorial Offices: 1600 John F. Kennedy Blvd., Ste. 1800, Philadelphia, PA 19103-2899. Customer Service Office: 3251 Riverport Lane, Maryland Heights, MO 63043. Periodicals postage paid at New York, NY and additional mailing offices. Subscription prices are $319.00 per year for US individuals, $640.00 per year for US institutions, $100.00 per year for US students and residents, $393.00 per year for Canadian individuals, $772.00 for Canadian institutions, $476.00 for international individuals, $772.00 per year for international institutions, $100.00 per year for Canadian students/residents, and $220.00 per year for foreign students/residents. To receive student/resident rate, orders must be accompanied by name of affiliated institution, date of term, and the *signature* of program/residency coordinator on institution letterhead. Orders will be billed at individual rate until proof of status is received. Foreign air speed delivery is included in all *Clinics* subscription prices. All prices are subject to change without notice. POSTMASTER: Send address changes to *Clinics in Podiatric Medicine and Surgery*, Elsevier Health Sciences Division, Subscription Customer Service, 3251 Riverport Lane, Maryland Heights, MO 63043. **Customer Service: 1-800-654-2452 (US). From outside of the US, call 314-447-8871. Fax: 314-447-8029. E-mail: JournalsCustomerService-usa@elsevier.com (for print support); JournalsOnlineSupport-usa@elsevier.com (for online support).**

Reprints. For copies of 100 or more of articles in this publication, please contact the Commercial Reprints Department, Elsevier Inc., 360 Park Avenue South, New York, NY 10010-1710. Tel.: 212-633-3874; Fax: 212-633-3820; E-mail: reprints@elsevier.com.

Clinics in Podiatric Medicine and Surgery is covered in *MEDLINE/PubMed (Index Medicus)* and *EMBASE/Excerpta Medica*.

Contributors

CONSULTING EDITOR

THOMAS J. CHANG, DPM
Clinical Professor and Past Chairman, Department of Podiatric Surgery, California College of Podiatric Medicine, Faculty, The Podiatry Institute, Redwood Orthopedic Surgery Associates, Santa Rosa, California

EDITOR

BYRON HUTCHINSON, DPM, FACFAS
Board of Directors, International Foot & Ankle Foundation, Board of Directors, Waldo Medical Foundation, Fellowship Director, CHI/Franciscan Advanced Foot & Ankle Fellowship, Franciscan Foot & Ankle Associates: Highline Clinic (Part of Franciscan Medical Group), Seattle, Washington

AUTHORS

MARIA BEGUM, DPM
Resident, Podiatric Medical Education, Our Lady of Lourdes Memorial Hospital, Graduate Medical Education, Binghamton, New York

SHIRLEY CHEN, DPM
Department of Plastic Surgery, Georgetown University School of Medicine, MedStar Washington Hospital Center Podiatric Surgery Residency, Center for Wound Healing, MedStar Georgetown University Hospital, Washington, DC

ALISON D'ANDELET, DPM, MHA
Attending Physician, Upper Chesapeake Medical Center, Bel Air, Maryland

LAWRENCE A. DIDOMENICO, DPM, FACFAS
Director of Residency Training, East Liverpool City Hospital, Director of Fellowship Training, NOMS Ankle and Foot Care Center

RACHEL GERBER, DPM
Resident, AMITA Health Saint Joseph Hospital Chicago, Chicago, Illinois

WILLIAM GRANT, DPM, MS, FACFAS
Tidewater Foot and Ankle, Virginia Beach, Virginia

LISA GRANT-McDONALD, DPM, AACFAS
Doctor, Tidewater Foot and Ankle, Virginia Beach, Virginia

STEPHANIE GUZELAK, DPM
Resident, Podiatric Medical Education, Our Lady of Lourdes Memorial Hospital, Graduate Medical Education, Binghamton, New York

LINDSEY R. HJELM, DPM
Podiatric Fellow, Department of Podiatry and Foot and Ankle Surgery, Virginia Mason Franciscan Health, Burien, Washington

BYRON HUTCHINSON, DPM, FACFAS
Board of Directors, International Foot & Ankle Foundation, Board of Directors, Waldo Medical Foundation, Fellowship Director, CHI/Franciscan Advanced Foot & Ankle Fellowship, Franciscan Foot & Ankle Associates: Highline Clinic (Part of Franciscan Medical Group), Seattle, Washington

GUIDO A. LAPORTA, DPM, MS, FACFAS
Director, Podiatric Medical Education, Our Lady of Lourdes Memorial Hospital, Binghamton, New York, USA

JOHN MARTUCCI, DPM, AACFAS
Fellow, NOMS Ankle and Foot Care Centers

JOHN D. MILLER, DPM
Department of Plastic Surgery, Georgetown University School of Medicine, MedStar Washington Hospital Center Podiatric Surgery Residency, Center for Wound Healing, MedStar Georgetown University Hospital, Washington, DC

KELSEY J. MILLONIG, DPM, MPH, AACFAS
Fellowship Trained Foot and Ankle Surgeon, East Village Foot & Ankle Surgeons, Des Moines, Iowa

STEPHANIE OEXEMAN, DPM, AACFAS, DABPM
Department of Surgery, Oexeman Foot and Ankle, PLLC, American Microsurgical Orthoplastic Society, Ascension Saint Joseph - Chicago, Chicago, Illinois

STEPHEN ROCKHILL, DPM
Resident, Franciscan Foot and Ankle Institute, Federal Way, Washington

EDGARDO R. RODRIGUEZ-COLLAZO, DPM
Director, CPME Postdoctoral Fellowship Complex Deformity Correction and Limb Reconstruction, Adults and Pediatric Ilizarov Limb Deformity Correction, Peripheral Nerve Reconstructive Microsurgery, Fellow, The Association of Extremity Nerve Surgeons, Founder, American Microsurgical Orthoplastic Society, Department of Surgery, Ascension Saint Joseph - Chicago, Laboure Outpatient Clinic, Chicago, Illinois

LAUREN L. SCHNACK, DPM, MS, AACFAS, FACPM
Fellow, CPME Postdoctoral Fellowship Complex Deformity Correction and Limb Reconstruction, American Microsurgical Orthoplastic Society, Ascension Saint Joseph - Chicago, Podiatric Fellow Office, Chicago, Illinois

MALLORY SCHWEITZER, DPM, MHA
Multicare Podiatry Associates, Tacoma, Washington

NOMAN A. SIDDIQUI, DPM, MHA, FACFAS
International Center for Limb Lengthening, Rubin Institute for Advanced Orthopedics, Sinai Hospital of Baltimore, Baltimore, Maryland; Department of Podiatry, Northwest Hospital, Randallstown, Maryland

HENRY D. SPINGOLA III, DPM, AACFAS
Fellow, NOMS Ankle and Foot Care Centers

JOHN S. STEINBERG, DPM, FACFAS
Professor, Department of Plastic Surgery, Georgetown University School of Medicine, Program Director, MedStar Washington Hospital Center Podiatric Surgery Residency, Co-Director, Center for Wound Healing, MedStar Georgetown University Hospital, Washington, DC

EMILY C. WAGLER, DPM
Attending Physician, Department of Podiatry and Foot and Ankle Surgery, The Vancouver Clinic, Vancouver, Washington

Contents

> Diabetes mellitus with the lack of glycemic control increases risks for developing comorbidities affecting organ systems responsible for critical function. The development of diabetic neuropathy predisposes patients to the onset of Charcot neuroarthropathy (CN). There is significant complexity with treatment of diabetic-induced CN, which can have an often delayed or missed diagnosis. Supervision and treatment from trained specialists are required to provide care for this multifaceted disease process. It is essential for patients to partner with glucose control, comorbidity prevention and care, as well as lower extremity management. Ultimately, CN can result in significant lower extremity deformity placing patients at risk of limb and life.

> Bone metabolism in the healthy, young adult is identified as a relatively stable process. Normal bone turnover is a dynamic state, which is conferred through intracellular signaling and complex cellular pathways. It has been well described in the literature that Charcot neuro-osteoarthropathy is a disease state, which is marked by intense bone turnover leading to structural collapse and dissolution of skeletal features of the foot and ankle. Within the last two decades, extensive interest has been placed in characterizing the metabolic pathogenesis of Charcot bone metabolism. Despite this work, there remains an incomplete understanding of this devastating disorder. In this article, we review bone histology, physiologic bone metabolism, biomarkers of bone metabolism, pathologic bone metabolism in Charcot diabetics, and potential avenues for intervention.

> Diabetic neuroarthropathy is a complication of diabetes mellitus that results in instability of the foot, structural deformity, and soft-tissue breakdown. Commonly, midfoot collapse of the medial, lateral, or both longitudinal arches may result in increased plantar pressures and subsequent midfoot ulceration. Many of these wounds can be successfully managed with local wound care and off-loading; however, surgical intervention becomes necessary in cases of osteomyelitis or when the wound

fails to heal despite conservative efforts. In cases where surgical reconstruction may not be indicated, nonreconstructive surgical efforts have
shown effectiveness in resolving wounds and allowing patients to return
to ambulatory lifestyles. This article serves as an update to current treatment recommendations for the nonreconstructive surgical management
of Charcot neuroarthropathy.

tThere are many similarities between nondiabetic and diabetic Charcot neuroarthropathy (CN) but many of the underlying causes causing nondiabetic
neuropathy and CN are associated with poor bone quality. Patient workup
for nondiabetic CN should include the underlying cause of the neuropathy
and optimization of bony healing, such as vitamin D supplementation and
bisphosphonate or calcitonin administration. Surgical reconstruction should
include the most robust fixation possible, as nondiabetic patients with CN
are more prone to delayed union.

Charcot can be a difficult clinical entity to diagnose in the acute phase, and
clinicians should have a high clinical suspicion in neuropathic patients who
present with erythema, edema, and warmth of the foot or ankle. Immobilization and nonweight-bearing should be immediately initiated when the
diagnosis of Charcot has been made and patients should remain
nonweight-bearing until the affected bones/joints have coalesced.
Educating patients and managing expectations is crucial to improve
compliance with the conservative treatment of Charcot and avoid the
long-term sequelae including severe deformity, ulceration and infection,
and amputation.

Reconstruction of the Charcot foot and ankle demonstrates significant
challenges to the foot and ankle surgeon. At present, there is limited clear
consensus on the best approach for preoperative optimization. The primary aim of Charcot reconstructions is to limit the risk of ulceration by
providing a stable plantigrade foot allowing ambulation. The focus of this
article is the discussion of modifiable risk factors associated with Charcot
reconstruction for preoperative optimization.

The Charcot diabetic foot presents unique challenges to the podiatric surgeon in the quest to salvage the limb. This disorder is an intersection of
prototypical metabolic diseases and neurodegenerative disorder. Furthermore, it can be considered a disease of bone and ligaments that is often
complicated by peripheral vascular disease and serious deep infection.
Presently, simplistic ablative surgical procedures and the brace-makers

art, still have a valid place in treating this disorder. Newer methods of surgical reconstruction are rapidly evolving to address distorted and nonfunctional limb. This article seeks to evidence the principles and practice of beaming the Charcot midfoot. As will be presented, the beam is a load-sharing device, which can be surgically introduced in an intramedullary method to restore architecture and strength to the Charcot foot. Problems with beam failure and migration have resulted in unsatisfactory outcomes as will be discussed. New Charcot-specific beams are currently reaching the podiatric surgeon with hopes of improving durability. In this article, we aim to address the surgical art of the beam, the engineering principles of beaming, and the novel introduction of a truss/tie rod configuration of beaming.

Charcot neuroarthropathy (CN) and its sequela is a disabling pathology in the foot and ankle. The 2-stage computer hexapod–assisted technique is an effective tool to address midfoot Charcot and ankle-hindfoot deformities to restore function and decrease the risk of amputation secondary to ulceration and infection. Although this is not the only technique available, it is an excellent option in cases with significant angular deformity or subluxation, need to reduce shortening of the foot, and in the presence of soft tissue defects, with or without concurrent soft tissue or bone infection.

Static circular fixation is a valuable tool for patients with Charcot foot and ankle deformities. The versatility of circular fixators allows for dynamic adjustments over time and can allow for off-loading of flaps or ulcers. The circular fixator can be used as a primary fixation device in cases of osteomyelitis or to facilitate lengthening when a segmental bone defect exists such as loss of the talus. As a secondary fixation device it can protect the internal fixation or be used when there is a compromised soft tissue envelope.

Hindfoot and ankle Charcot neuroarthropathy is a challenging condition to treat, specifically with segmental bone defects secondary to avascular necrosis or infection. Several techniques exist alongside continued challenges of nonunion and complication rates. The authors assert that combining distal tibial distraction osteogenesis with external fixation in tibiocalcaneal or tibiotalocalcaneal arthrodesis should be considered an effective method for management of complex Charcot neuroarthropathy conditions of the ankle. This staged procedure technique resulted in a high rate of union in patients who are often considered a high risk for nonunion, as well as eradication of infection, minimal soft tissue disruption, and improvement in limb length.

Surgical reconstruction of Charcot arthropathy in the foot and ankle is extremely difficult. The fundamentals of reconstruction are necessary to provide adequate outcome. Removing and resecting the diseased bone is needed along with good anatomic alignment and rigid fixation. This reconstructive surgery is not only difficult from medical management point of view but also involves patient compliance and good technical components of the surgery from the surgeon. The surgeon must have skills with internal and external fixation, a good understanding of lower extremity vascular disease, and a good understanding of infectious disease and plastic surgical techniques of the lower extremity.

Approximately 20% of patients with diabetic peripheral neuropathy (DPN) endorse painful sensations such as prickling, stabbing, and burning pain that reflect small-fiber involvement. Although glycemic control is crucial to delay the onset and progression of DPN, there have been many reports on the use of decompression nerve surgery to aid in the treatment of DPN.

CLINICS IN PODIATRIC MEDICINE AND SURGERY

Foreword

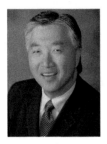

Thomas J. Chang, DPM
Consulting Editor

The neuropathic Charcot foot has been a fascinating disease process to study throughout my whole career. As a resident, I remember scrubbing in many cases of Charcot reconstruction with Drs McGlamry, Ruch, Kalish, and Banks in 1989–1993. Drs McGlamry and Ruch started this journey into Charcot reconstruction in the mid-1980s, and this was always done while the foot was in the quiescent phase of disease. A Charcot reconstruction was always an open Achilles tendon lengthening and open surgical stabilization of the involved areas of bone injury. Rocker bottom feet were converted into feet with visible arches, involving a variety of metal fixation and prolonged cast immobilization. At that time, there were no external fixation constructs, no concepts of intramedullary beaming, and rarely, biologics.

We have evolved a tremendous amount since those days. Extensive research and clinical experiences have dramatically improved the medical and surgical management of neuropathic osteoarthropathy. Medically, we better understand the biochemical pathways involved, implementing bone supportive therapies and higher sensitivity and specificity with medical imaging and the timing of surgery.

Surgical outcomes have equally improved with further understanding of biomechanical principles. This includes dynamic functional control of the medial and lateral columns, consideration of ankle and hindfoot contributions, and a continuing enhancement of fixation constructs.

Dr Hutchinson has extensively studied the neuropathic foot and ankle over the past 25 years. He has taken inspiration from many before him and has become a modern pioneer of many concepts applied to this growing discussion. I applaud his dedication and passion into this area and his willingness to share this body of knowledge with the foot and ankle community.

Clin Podiatr Med Surg 39 (2022) xiii–xiv
https://doi.org/10.1016/j.cpm.2022.08.001
0891-8422/22/© 2022 Published by Elsevier Inc.

These are extremely difficult patients, and this is an invaluable contribution to continue the discussion. I hope you enjoy this issue.

Thomas J. Chang, DPM
Redwood Orthopedic Surgery Associates
208 Concourse Boulevard
Santa Rosa, CA 95403, USA

E-mail address:
thomaschang14@comcast.net

Preface

Current Concepts in Charcot Neuroarthropathy

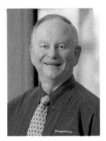

Byron Hutchinson, DPM, FACFAS
Editor

Charcot neuroarthropathy (CN) is a complex and difficult problem to manage on any level. The management of CN has evolved significantly since the first description of this debilitating condition. The proper evaluation and consideration of the appropriate reconstructive options can allow patients to walk with a plantigrade foot, increase their quality of life, and decrease morbidity. The advancements in the management of this condition in the past two decades have been extraordinary. Successful limb salvage owes much to this forward thinking and to the courage, patience, and skills of the physicians and surgeons who manage this challenging population.

No problem can withstand the assault of sustained thinking

—Voltaire

I think this quote from Voltaire summarizes this perfectly. No one gets through life on one's own, and clearly this applies to the practice of medicine and surgery as well. Treating CN, for me personally, has been both a rewarding and a humbling experience. My approach to CN has evolved through the years of education, reflection, and collaboration with multidisciplinary mentors and colleagues, and I would like to take this opportunity to thank each and every one of them.

This issue of *Clinics in Podiatric Medicine and Surgery* brings together the latest concepts about managing the Charcot patient from the best minds in the field. I am extremely proud to present this publication and want to thank each contributor for the time, effort, and expertise. My hope is that this issue provides a framework for

Clin Podiatr Med Surg 39 (2022) xv–xvi
https://doi.org/10.1016/j.cpm.2022.07.001
0891-8422/22/© 2022 Published by Elsevier Inc.

physicians interested in CN, stimulates further conversation, forges new concepts, and improves treatment options for this difficult and challenging condition.

Byron Hutchinson, DPM, FACFAS
Franciscan Foot & Ankle Associates:
Highline Clinic
16233 Sylvester Road SW G-10
Seattle, WA 98166, USA

E-mail address:
highlinef@aol.com

Diabetes Mellitus
An Overview in Relationship to Charcot Neuroarthropathy

Lindsey R. Hjelm, DPM

KEYWORDS

- Diabetes mellitus • Type 1 diabetes • Type 2 diabetes • Charcot neuroarthropathy
- Neuropathy • Ulceration

KEY POINTS

- The prevalence of diabetes mellitus has continued to increase at alarming rates during the past 4 decades. Continued public health efforts are being made to reduce the incidence and improve treatment worldwide.
- There are multiple comorbidities associated with diabetes that can significantly influence patient health as well as increase predisposition for Charcot neuroarthropathy (CN).
- CN is most commonly caused by diabetes mellitus in the setting of neuropathy. There are many challenges encountered with treatment, particularly in the presence of ulceration.

DIABETES MELLITUS: AN OVERVIEW

There are approximately 463 million adults living with diabetes mellitus worldwide, which is a significant increase from the 108 million reported by the World Health Organization (WHO) in 1980 and 422 million in 2014.[1,2] It has been reported that most people with this condition are found within low-income and middle-income countries.[2] Although resources may be available in communities, there is concern about methods of delivery and distribution. As a result, there is a lack of implemented services regarding education, prevention, and evidence-based treatment of individuals with diabetes. In North America, data published by the WHO in 2021 reported 11.7% prevalence of diabetes, higher than any other region or continent. Within this diabetic population, 75.4% had an HbA1c less than 8%. As prevalence increases, there will be continued catastrophic impact to communities worldwide suffering from diabetes mellitus.[3]

Diabetes mellitus is a disorder of the endocrine system that ultimately affects the whole body. There are two types of diabetes, Type-1 (T1) and Type-2 (T2), which

Department of Podiatry and Foot & Ankle Surgery, Virginia Mason Franciscan Health, 16233 Sylvester Road SW G-10, Burien, WA 98166, USA
E-mail address: lindseyhjelm@gmail.com

Clin Podiatr Med Surg 39 (2022) 535–542
https://doi.org/10.1016/j.cpm.2022.05.001
0891-8422/22/© 2022 Elsevier Inc. All rights reserved.

have similarities and differences outlined in greater detail below. Diagnosis of diabetes is determined with fasting blood glucose level greater than 126 mg/dL, random blood glucose concentration of 200 mg/dL, or oral glucose intolerance test. Of interest in this publication is the relationship between diabetes mellitus and the development of peripheral neuropathy leading to Charcot neuroarthropathy (CN).

TYPE 1

T1 diabetes has demonstrated annual increases in incidence of 2% to 3% per year.[4] Although commonly understood as an autoimmune disorder in which beta cells are destroyed by T cells, new research is guiding developments in pathophysiology. Genetic contributions have been seen as a primary cause; however, there is evidence to suggest environmental and behavioral factors are influencing increased incidence in T1 diabetes as well. Genetic factors have long been studied siting commonly inherited human leukocyte antigen alleles within family members who have T1 diabetes. However, new studies are showing a lack of genetic material predisposing patients. Further research is being performed to discover the multifaceted and complex interplay of individuals to their environment, microbiome, metabolism, and immune system.[5]

Symptom presentation can differ in T1 diabetic patients as well as age range. In children, symptom presentation includes polyuria, polydipsia, and weight loss, whereas in adults, there is more variability.[5] Although T1 diabetes is commonly classified as juvenile onset, there are 50% of cases that do not present until adulthood.[6] Careful considerations should be made for adult onset because there can be misdiagnoses of contrasting disease process of T2 diabetes.[7] The disease course results in progressive loss of functional pancreatic beta cells from self-inflicted T cells; however, there is not complete loss of beta cells, which allows for microsecretion of C peptide.[8] According to the Diabetes Control and Complications Trial, continued C peptide secretion reduces the development of retinopathy, nephropathy, and hypoglycemia.[9] The preventative power of continued secretion of C peptide could reduce risks associated with comorbidities affiliated with diabetes. The best prevention for associated health conditions with diabetes includes management of blood glucose with insulin. Further research is being performed to assist with preservation and restoration of beta cells, which could be instrumental treatment and prevention.

TYPE 2

In contrast to T1 diabetes, T2 diabetes can have multiple disturbances in glucose homeostasis. There is impaired insulin secretion, tissue resistance to insulin, as well as inhibition in splanchnic glucose uptake.[10] During disease progression, T2 diabetics demonstrate twice the plasma insulin concentration to that of their healthy age-matched controls, which is in response to decreased tissue sensitization to insulin. There is a cyclic pattern of hyperinsulemia and peripheral tissue resistance, both of which causing beta cells to eventually deteriorate with inability to maintain demands for insulin production.[11] This becomes a vicious cycle that without significant lifestyle modifications can progress rapidly and negatively affect multiple organ systems.

Increased life span of aging populations in conjunction with reduced activity and poor diet has influenced the prevalence observed of T2 diabetes worldwide.[12] In adults, prevalence has almost doubled from 1980 to 2014.[2] Correlation of T2 diabetes with sedentary lifestyle and Western-based diet have been strongly associated. The Western diet has become more widely available across the planet with increased carbohydrate consumption and sweetened beverages. Beyond poor sources of nutrition, there are additional factors including poor sleep hygiene, increased stress, depression as well as socioeconomic factors that may be lesser known.[13] Individuals that engage in moderate-to-high intensity activity, increased consumption of plant-based foods, active social network, and reduced smoking or alcohol intake are less likely to develop the disease.[14,15] Overall, the greatest protective factor against T2 diabetes is the reduction and prevention of ectopic fat. Glucose homeostasis improves even the first week after a bariatric surgery or application of a low calorie diet.[16,17] These lifestyle modifications need to be routinely presented to patients for preventative and treatment options.

COMORBIDITIES AND HEALTH RISKS ASSOCIATED WITH DIABETES

Diabetes mellitus has been known to accelerate the formation of other health-related comorbidities, such as systemic disease related to the peripheral vascular, cardiovascular, kidney, and peripheral neuropathy. Because of diabetes, these organ systems can suffer, deteriorate, or completely fail. The synergistic effects of diabetes and hypertension have resulted in cardiovascular disease being the leading cause of death in T2 diabetic.[18] Compared with the general population, hypertension is diagnosed alongside diabetes at alarming rates and occurs in most T2 patients.[18] The affects of uncontrolled hypertension can result in significant large and small vessel disease. Due to the presence of hypertension and hyperglycemia, remodeling of arterial walls results in increased rigidity and narrowing.[19] Comparatively, with T1 diabetics, a foundational study performed by Diabetes Control and Complication Trial outlined that proper glucose management can lead to a reduction in microvascular and cardiovascular complications.[20] There has not been significant genetic relationships associated with T1 diabetes and cardiovascular complications; however, patient profiles such as female gender and low income and education demonstrate high risks of both macro and microvascular complications.[21,22] Through improved utilization of screening, treatment, and glucose control, WHO suggests that greater than 40% of cardiovascular related deaths can be avoided.[3]

Another common comorbidity is kidney disease, which is most commonly caused by diabetes mellitus. The duration of diabetes, the presence of hypertension, and level of glycemic control are risk factors for the development of nephropathy.[23] It has been estimated that 30% of T1 diabetics and 40% of T2 diabetics will develop chronic kidney disease.[24] The incidence of disease in accompaniment with diabetes is high; however, these values have decreased during the last 20 years secondary to increased efforts for screening, prevention, and treatment.[25] Kidney disease can lead to metabolic derangement because of increased filtration secondary to efferent arteriole vasoconstriction, and oxidative stresses. Without proper treatment, the disease can progress leading to increased morbidity and mortality with nearly 20% of diabetics requiring dialysis in the United States.[26]

Finally, and of greatest impact to the development of CN, neuropathy often accompanies diabetes and can result in significant disability. It impairs balance, sensory loss, gait instability, falls, as well as ulceration and amputation. Diabetes is the most commonly caused by neuropathy and 20% of diabetics have neuropathy on initial diagnoses.[27] Stino and colleagues describe that diabetic neuropathy differs from cryptogenic peripheral neuropathy that develops in nondiabetics. However, in some cases T2 diabetics can develop both cryptogenic and well as standard diabetic neuropathy putting them at further risk for CN. Although there are medications to assist with discomfort, there are no curative treatments for this condition. In T1 diabetics, the best prevention is aggressive glycemic control. Loss of protective sensation with diabetic neuropathy places significant risk on patients for developing ulcerations. These can develop based on pressure, friction, deformity, and repeated microtrauma that remain undetected by patients. The presence of neuropathy risks the development of CN. Diabetic-induced CN that present with ulcerations are 6 to 12 times more prone to amputation.[28,29] Additionally, mortality rates are nearly three times higher in patients with CN[30]; however, this risk if still lower than that of diabetics who develop a foot ulcer.[31,32]

DIABETES AND RELATIONSHIP WITH CHARCOT NEUROARTHOPATHY

Diabetes mellitus is the most common cause of CN. The incidence and prevalence of CN in diabetics ranges from 0.1% to 0.4%[33] and as high as 29% in those with peripheral neuropathy.[34] A study performed by Petrova outlined characteristics of T1 diabetics at high risk for developing CN, and this included middle-aged, long-standing diabetics with lack of glucose control and morbid obesity.[35–37] Aside from poor glucose control, Samann evaluated 164 patients with diabetic nephropathy and outlined that having a high level of microalbuminuria may be a factor to predict the development of CN. Thus hypotehsizing that microalbuminuria may be more sensitive than the level of HbA1c control predicting the onset of CN.[38] Although CN exclusively develops in the presence of neuropathy, the prevalence in diabetics still remains relatively low. Other neurologic conditions with associated neuropathy have also been cited such as leprosy, alcoholic neuropathy, tabes dorsals, syringomyelia, or syphilis to name a few.[39] Another contributing factor associated with diabetics developing CN is related to gait modifications from chronic hyperglycemia and glycoslylation of lower extremity tendons. Because intrinsic musculature atrophies, there is imbalance of extrinsic musculature leading to digital deformities. Additionally, glycosylation specifically of the Achilles tendon leads to stiffness and shortening, which results in equinus.[40] Patients are forced to spend increased time in stance phase as well as exert increased plantar pressures.[41] Increased loading or stress on a neuropathic foot can lead to a proinflammatory state contributing to CN. Other predisposing factors of CN development include history of ulceration, trauma, and renal transplant. Individuals that are diabetic and demonstrate any of these risk factors should be closely monitored by a trained foot and ankle specialist.

Although the exact pathophysiology associated with Charcot development is not fully known, the presence of neuropathy and inflammation leads to osteoclastogenesis. This can result in progressive deformity with fracturing, resorption, and dislocation of the weight-bearing bones in the lower extremity. There needs to be a high suspicion for CN by primary providers and specialists due to the severity and potential progression of the disease with continued weight bearing on a compromised limb.[42] Often it has been cited that CN is underdiagnosed or carries a delayed diagnosis that can be detrimental to patients who have an unstable limb.[43]

Initial presentation of CN is consistent with a red, hot, swollen extremity. Within a diabetic patient, there are multiple diagnoses that may present similarly such as cellulitis, osteomyelitis, or gout to name a few. However, this should warrant immediate evaluation for suspected CN. A recent traumatic event such as an ankle or foot sprain could also represent a Charcot event with inflammatory changes causing joint instability. Often these clinical scenarios do not warrant radiographic imaging; however, suspicion of CN can be pivotal to diagnosis. Aside from radiographic findings, which may be initially subtle, the presence of a wound, elevated C-reactive protein or erythrocyte sedimentation rate can also be diagnostic.[44] Increased inflammatory markers are also present with infection; however, to differentiate from infections, CN usually does not present with increased blood glucose, increased insulin requirements, or decreased glucose control as infection does. Other strategies of diagnoses are contralateral limb temperature difference of 2°, foot instability, or the ability to have swelling resolve with elevation, which indicates CN.[45,46] Prompt diagnosis is essential for halting the progressive disease course, which can lead to the risk of limb loss. CN commonly presents unilaterally but as patients seek treatment of one extremity, anticipated increases in contralateral limb weight bearing can cause further precipitation of CN.[41]

CN in the diabetic patient is particularly vulnerable to progressive disease process due to fragile bone. Histologic studies have outlined that CN bone has characteristics of reactive bone that is woven in appearance and structurally immature. Therefore, the combination of CN with diabetes demonstrates bone with decreased cellular components, inhibition of cellular repair leading, and ultimately can lead to greater osseous damage.[47] Contrasting from these concerns outlined by La Fontaine, there have been studies demonstrating osseous protective effects of insulin and metformin, which can inhibit apoptosis or suppression of osseous cell lines.[48–50]

Cates and colleagues performed a comparison study between diabetics and nondiabetics who received CN reconstructive procedures. It determined that nondiabetic patients with CN were 17.6 times more likely to ambulate postoperatively and 16.4 times at greater risk of developing a delayed union compared with diabetics.[51] Factors most strongly associated with diabetics not returning to ambulation include severity of neuropathy, peripheral vascular disease, cardiovascular disease, and renal failure.[52] Based on previous concerns related to diabetic bone quality in combination with Charcot, Cates and colleagues determined decreased bone mineral density was more commonly found in nondiabetics due to causes of neuropathy that require treatment with steroids, HIV, alcohol abuse, and chemotherapy. Although patients with nondiabetic CN may have a greater rate of ambulation after reconstruction, the underlying cause of CN could affect osseous capabilities to heal. Although both groups in Cates study had neuropathy, the diabetic group was more likely to have ulcerations. The presence of ulcerations has been determined to be the greatest precipitant of CN compared with other comorbidities or demographics.[51] Difficulty for diabetics returning to ambulation could also be related to preoperative ulcerations leading to infection, further bone resection, and ultimately causing greater change as well as instability of foot.[52–55] Treatment of Diabetic CN requires diligent management during all phases of care starting with prompt diagnosis, glycemic control, off-loading deformities, and surgical care.

There is significant complexity regarding the management of diabetes with CN. Challenges in treatment are encountered with accompanied comorbidities such as cardiovascular and kidney disease. The presence of neuropathy with ulcerations puts diabetic patients at increased risk for the development of CN and complications. Continued worldwide public health efforts are needed to reduce prevalence of diabetes. Lifestyle changes, education, and treatment adherence are important aspects of patient care that are required to maximize health of diabetic patients.

CLINICS CARE POINTS

- Do not overlook lower extremity swelling, warmth or redness in a neuropathic patient, have a high suspicion for CN and proceed with getting weight bearing radiographic imaging.

- While diabetes is the most common cause of neuropathic conditions, recognize there are many other sources that can lead to CN.

- A partnering relationship between lower extremity, primary care and endocrine specialists can be essential for delivery limb preserving treatments successfully.

DISCLOSURES

The author has nothing to disclose.

REFERENCES

1. International Diabetes Federation. IDF diabetes atlas. 2019. Available at: www. diabetesatlas.org. Accessed October 20, 2021.
2. NDC Risk Factor Collaboration. Worldwide trends in diabetes since 1980: a pooled analysis of 751 population-based studies with 4.4 million participants. Lancet 2016;387:1513–30.
3. Gregg E, Buckley J, Ali M, et al. J improving health outcomes of people with diabetes mellitus: target setting to reduce the global burden of diabetes mellitus by 2030. World Health Organization; 2021. Accessed. https://www.who.int/.
4. Maahs DM, West NA, Lawrence JM, et al. Epidemiology of type 1 diabetes. Endocrinol Metab Clin North Am 2010;39:481–97.
5. DiMeglio LA, Evans-Molina C, Oram RA. Type 1 diabetes. The Lancet 2018; 391(10138):2449–62.
6. Thomas NJ, Jones SE, Weedon MN, et al. Frequency and phenotype of type 1 diabetes in the first six decades of life: a cross-sectional, genetically stratified survival analysis from UK Biobank. Lancet Diabetes Endocrinol 2018;6:122–9.
7. Hope SV, Wienand-Barnett S, Shepherd M, et al. Practical classification guidelines for diabetes in patients treated with insulin: a cross-sectional study of the accuracy of diabetes diagnosis. Br J Gen Pract 2016;66:e315–22.
8. Davis AK, DuBose SN, Haller MJ, et al. Prevalence of detectable C-peptide according to age at diagnosis and duration of type 1 diabetes. Diabetes Care 2015;38:476–81.
9. Zenz S, Mader JK, Regittnig W, et al. Impact of C-peptide status on the response of glucagon and endogenous glucose production to induced hypoglycaemia in T1DM. J Clin Endocrinol Metab 2018;103:1408–17.
10. DeFronzo RA. Pathogenesis of type 2 diabetes mellitus. Med Clin North Am 2004; 88(4):787–835.
11. DeFronzo RA. Pathogenesis of type 2 diabetes mellitus: metabolic and molecular implications for identifying diabetes genes. Diabetes 1997;5:177–269.
12. Chatterjee S, Khunti K, Davies MJ. Type 2 diabetes. Lancet 2017;389(10085): 2239–51.
13. Kolb H, Martin S. Environmental/lifestyle factors in the pathogenesis and prevention of type 2 diabetes. BMC Med 2017;15(1):131.
14. Shadyab AH, LaCroix AZ. Genetic factors associated with longevity: a review of recent findings. Ageing Res Rev 2015;19:1–7.
15. Loef M, Walach H. The combined effects of healthy lifestyle behaviors on all cause mortality: a systematic review and meta-analysis. Prev Med 2012;55: 163–70.
16. Lim EL, Hollingsworth KG, Aribisala BS, et al. Reversal of type 2 diabetes: normalisation of beta cell function in association with decreased pancreas and liver triacylglycerol. Diabetologia 2011;54:2506–14.
17. Nguyen KT, Korner J. The sum of many parts: potential mechanisms for improvement in glucose homeostasis after bariatric surgery. Curr Diab Rep 2014;14:481.
18. Strain WD, Paldánius PM. Diabetes, cardiovascular disease and the microcirculation. Cardiovasc Diabetol 2018;17:57. https://doi.org/10.1186/s12933-018-0703-2.

19. Smulyan H, Lieber A, Safar ME. Hypertension, diabetes type II, and their association: role of arterial stiffness. Am J Hypertens 2016;29:5–13.
20. Nathan DM. The diabetes control and complications trial/epidemiology of diabetes interventions and complications study at 30 years: overview. Diabetes Care 2014;37:9–16.
21. Huxley RR, Peters SA, Mishra GD, et al. Risk of all-cause mortality and vascular events in women versus men with type 1 diabetes: a systematic review and meta-analysis. Lancet Diabetes Endocrinol 2015;3:198–206.
22. Secrest AM, Costacou T, Gutelius B, et al. Associations between socioeconomic status and major complications in type 1 diabetes: the Pittsburgh epidemiology of diabetes complication (EDC) study. Ann Epidemiol 2011;21:374–81.
23. Adler AI, Stevens RJ, Manley SE, et al. Development and progression of nephropathy in type 2 diabetes: the United Kingdom Prospective Diabetes Study (UKPDS 64). Kidney Int 2003;63(1):225–32.
24. United States Renal Data System. 2018 USRDS annual data report: CKD in the general population. Bethesda, MD: United States Renal Data System; 2018. p. 1–28.
25. Bonner R, Albajrami O, Hudspeth J, et al. Diabetic kidney disease. Primary care: clinics in office practice 2020. https://doi.org/10.1016/j.pop.2020.08.004.
26. United States Renal Data System. USRDS Annual Data Report: incidence, prevalence, patient characteristics, and treatment modalities. Am J Kidney Dis 2018; 59(1 SUPPL. 1). https://doi.org/10.1053/j.ajkd.2011.10.027.
27. Stino AM, Smith AG. Peripheral neuropathy in prediabetes and the metabolic syndrome. J Diabetes Invest 2017;8(5):646–55.
28. Sohn M-W, Todd AL, Stuck RM, et al. Mortality risk of Charcot arthropathy compared with that of diabetic foot ulcer and diabetes alone. Diabetes Care 2009;32(5):816–21.
29. Wukich DK, Sadoskas D, Vaudreuil NJ, et al. Comparison of diabetic Charcot patients with and without foot wounds. Foot Ankle Int 2017;38:140–8.
30. Armstrong DG, Todd WF, Lavery LA, et al. The natural history of acute Charcot's arthropathy in a diabetic foot specialty clinic. Diabet Med 1997;14:357–63.
31. Chaudhry S, Bhansali A, Rastogi A. Mortality in Asian Indians with Charcot's neuroarthropathy: a nested cohort prospective study. Acta Diabetol 2019;56(12): 1259–64.
32. Sohn MW, Stuck RM, Pinzur M, et al. Lower-extremity amputation risk after Charcot arthropathy and diabetic foot ulcer. Diabetes Care 2009;33:98–100.
33. Dardari D. An overview of Charcot's neuroarthropathy. J Clin Translational Endocrinol 2020;22:100239.
34. Cofield R, Motrisin M, Beabout J. Diabetic neuroarthropathy in the foot: patient characteristics and patterns of radiographic changes. Foot Ankle Int 1983; 4:5–22.
35. Petrova NL, Edmonds ME. Acute Charcot neuro-osteoarthropathy. Diabetes Metab Res Rev 2016;32:281–6.
36. Gouveri E. Charcot osteoarthropathy in diabetes: a brief review with an emphasis on clinical practice. World J Diabetes 2011;2(5):59–65.
37. Game FL, Catlow R, Jones GR, et al. Audit of acute Charcot's disease in the UK: the CDUK study. Diabetologia 2012;55(1):32–5.
38. Samann A, Pofahl S, Lehmann T, et al. Diabetic nephropathy but not HbA1c is predictive for frequent complications of Charcot feet - long-term follow-up of 164 consecutive patients with 195 acute Charcot feet. Exp Clin Endocrinol Diabetes 2012;120(6):335–9.

39. Frykberg R, Belczyk R. Epidemiology of the Charcot foot. Clin Podiatr Med Surg 2008;25(1):17–28.
40. Grant WP, Sullivan R, Sonenshine DE, et al. Electron microscopic investigation of the effects of diabetes mellitus on the Achilles tendon. J Foot Ankle Surg 1997;36: 272–8.
41. Armstrong DG, Lavery LA. Elevated peak plantar pressures in patients who have Charcot arthropathy. J Bone Jt Surg Br 1998;80A:365–9.
42. Varma AK. Charcot neuroarthropathy of the foot and ankle: a review. J Foot Ankle Surg 2013;52(6):740–9.
43. Kavitha KV, Patil VS, Sanjeevi CB, et al. New concepts in the management of Charcot neuroarthropathy in diabetes. Adv Exp Med Biol 2020;1307:391–415.
44. Loredo R, Rahal A, Garcia G, et al. Imaging of the diabetic foot diagnostic dilemmas. Foot Ankle Spec 2010;3(5):249–64.
45. Assal M, Stern R. Realignment and extended fusion with use of a medial column screw midfoot deformities secondary to diabetic neuropathy. J Bone Jt Surg Am 2009;91:812–20.
46. Madan SS, Pai DR. Charcot neuroarthropathy of the foot and ankle. Orthop Surg 2013;5(2):86–93.
47. La Fontaine J, Shibuya N, Sampson W, et al. Trabecular quality and cellular characteristics of nor- mal, diabetic, and Charcot bone. J Foot Ankle Surg 2011;50(6): 648–53.
48. Zheng L, Shen X, Ye J, et al. Metformin alleviates hyperglycemia- induced apoptosis and differentiation suppression in osteoblasts through inhibiting the TLR4 signaling pathway. Life Sci 2019;216:29–38.
49. Marycz K, Tomaszewski KA, Kornicka K, et al. Metformin decreases reactive oxygen species, enhances osteogenic properties of adipose-derived multipotent mesenchymal stem cells in vitro, and increases bone density in vivo. Oxidative Med Cell Longevity 2016;2016:1–19.
50. Attinger CE, Brown BJ. Amputation and ambulation in diabetic patients: function is the goal. Diabetes/Metabolism Res Rev 2012;28:93–6.
51. Cates NK, Wagler EC, Bunka TJ, et al. Charcot reconstruction: outcomes in patients with and without diabetes. J Foot Ankle Surg 2020;59(6):1229–33.
52. Fauzi AA, Chung TY, Latif LA. Risk factors of diabetic foot Charcot arthropathy: a case-control study at a Malaysian tertiary care center. Singapore Med J 2016;57: 198–203.
53. Kanade RV, Van Deursen RW, Harding KG, et al. Investigation of standing balance in patients with diabetic neuropathy at different stages of foot complications. Clin Biomech 2008;23:1183–91.
54. Li T, He S, Liu S, et al. Effects of different exercise durations on Keap1-Nrf2-ARE pathway activation in mouse skeletal muscle. Free Radic Res 2015;49:1269–74.
55. Stevens MJ, Edmonds ME, Foster AV, et al. Selective neuropathy and preserved vascular responses in the diabetic Charcot foot. Diabetologia 1992;35:148–54.

Bone Metabolism in Charcot

Lisa Grant-McDonald, DPM, AACFAS*, William Grant, DPM, FACFAS

KEYWORDS

- Charcot foot • Diabetic neuropathic osteoarthropathy • Pathogenesis
- Receptor activator of nuclear factor k-β ligand (RANKL)

KEY POINTS

- The pathogenesis of Charcot neuropathic osteoarthropathy is a constellation of pathways that abnormally entice inflammation, accentuate bone lysis, and inhibit bone formation.
- Bone metabolism studies in the Charcot population are often descriptive in nature and rarely link markers of bone turnover to causation.
- Pathway-targeted therapy has shown some success in reducing bone turnover in acute phase patients.

CHARCOT BONE STRUCTURE AND CELL TYPE

Bone metabolism and healing is a highly reserved and complex process that involves thousands of genes to function in a very coordinated manner.[1] Failure of any of these processes can result in delayed union or nonunion, producing a tissue that is mechanically and structurally insufficient.[2] Bone is a form of matrix dense connective tissue that has been mineralized by calcium phosphate resulting in a rigid state. The body's skeleton acts to provide structure, shape, and allows for locomotion.[3]

Two chief histologic types of mature bone exist: cortical and trabecular. Cortical bone is the densely packed and well-structured bone, which is most abundantly found in long bones and as the surface layer of flat bones.[4] Cortical bone is well organized into concentric patterns known as lamella that forms around a central Haversian canal. This system aids in nutrient acquisition and intracellular communication between osteocytes, a terminally differentiated bone cell that functions in calcium homeostasis.[1,2] The other chief type of bone is trabecular bone, which is significantly less organized. Trabecular bone forms extensions or a honeycomb pattern called trabeculae that form along lines of stress. The two principal cell types are dispersed dependent on the structural needs (compression vs shear force) of the resultant bone.[5]

Newly formed trabecular bone undergoes stabilization by the cross-linking of collagen fibers. Cross-links can form from the enzymatic process through the action of lysyl oxidase or nonenzymatically via advanced glycation end products (AGEs). The degree of

---

Tidewater Foot and Ankle, 760 Independence Boulevard, Virginia Beach, VA 23455, USA
* Corresponding author.
E-mail address: lisa.m.grantmcdonald@gmail.com

Clin Podiatr Med Surg 39 (2022) 543–557
https://doi.org/10.1016/j.cpm.2022.05.002
0891-8422/22/© 2022 Elsevier Inc. All rights reserved.

podiatric.theclinics.com

cross-linking in a healthy person is determined by the mechanical need of the bone. Nonenzymatic cross-linking is a by-product of oxidative stress and normal aging.[6]

PHYSIOLOGIC BONE METABOLISM

The rate of physiologic bone turnover is quite rapid, with 5% to 7% of bone mass recycled every week.[4] Bone turnover can occur in both cancellous and cortical bone. Typically, bones are composed of an outer cortical layer encasing the cancellous bone. Cortical bone has two interfaces: periosteal (outer surface) that is continuous with the periosteum and the endosteal (inner surface) that is in communication with the cancellous bone. The most common site of bone turnover is from the endosteal (internal) surface and is coordinated by osteoblasts (bone-forming cells) and osteoclasts (bone destruction cells).[1] The most basic entities of bone metabolism are osteocytes, osteoblasts, and osteoclasts that are signaled by hormones, mechanical forces, and cytokines to function in a very synchronized process. Most of the processes are mediated by osteocytes, which are primarily signaled by local stimuli to release metalloproteinase to degrade the tissue matrix.[1,2,4]

Osteoclasts are specialized multinucleated giant cells whose primary function is to resorb bone. Osteoclasts are derived from an undifferentiated monocyte origin and undergo four stages of maturation. This immunehistologic origin may explain why bone metabolism is affected so intensely by an immune-compromised state. The process of differentiation into mature osteoclast is initiated through cell-to-cell signaling. Once differentiated, the mature osteocyte closely associates with the bone surface and uses the "ruffled border" to bind to the bone's matrix adhesion proteins.[4] Here, the ruffled border seals to the bone surface to form Howship's lacunae, or an acidic pit that solubilizes minerals and degrades the bone. Osteoclast recruitment, differentiation, and function are tightly regulated through communication with osteoblasts using various molecular signals. The suggested life span of an osteoclast is a range of 2 to 6 weeks. Following the liberation of calcium and the completed function of bone degradation, it is thought that osteoclasts undergo preprogramed cellular apoptosis. New research, however, has identified an alternative cell fate in which osteoclast derivatives remain as a primed substrate to reactivate fusion and differentiation of other precursor cells.[4] This new pathway provides the possibility of breakaway osseous destruction; however, further research is required to substantiate these findings.

Osteoblasts play an essential role in bone remodeling by depositing collagen scaffold (osteoid) and regulating osteoclastogenesis and bone resorption. Osteoblast cell origin is mesenchymal stem cells that undergo differentiation. Osteoblasts are attracted to the endosteal surface to form new osteoid, which will later be calcified. They produce much of the required building blocks of bone including type I collagen, macrophage-colony stimulating factor, glycosaminoglycan, proteoglycans, glycoproteins (osteocalcin and osteopontin), and alkaline phosphatase. The osteoblast cell fate is to be surrounded by calcified osteoid and mature into osteocytes. Mature osteocytes are considered the basic unit of bone. The osteocyte network regulates cell-to-cell signaling and identifies local environmental needs.[4] A great body of research has identified the unique pathways of cell signaling, differentiation of osteogenic precursors, and the ultimate terminal state of bone cells. This article focuses specifically on the pathways that have been described in Charcot pathophysiology.

PHYSIOLOGIC BONE SIGNALING

Much like the rest of the body, the peripheral nervous system is what relays stimuli between the central nervous system (CNS) and the bone. The nerves of the skeleton are a mix between unmyelinated and myelinated, small and medium diameter fibers, and are capable of sensing sympathetic and parasympathetic messages. The sensory nerves of the skeleton relay information regarding pain, pressure, and other stimuli to and from the bone. The bone then uses these signals to respond via anabolic or catabolic pathways.[7]

Nervous tissue enters the bone through Haversian systems where they are able to engage in local metabolism. Surprisingly, no true synapse has been identified in bone and instead cellular messaging occurs via non-synaptic vesicular fusion release of neurotransmitters within the extracellular space. These neurotransmitters are then able to engage with local bone cells to produce the intended end result.[7,8] Studies have acknowledged several important neurotransmitters involved in bone cell signaling including calcific gene-related peptide (CGRP), substance P (SP), norepinephrine, and neuropeptide Y. It is important to note that numerous tissue cells throughout the body actively express each of these neurotransmitters.[9,10] Often the interpretations made during in vitro studies are performed in isolation and may not replicate the actual function of these processes.

Much of the efferent or local bone stimulation is a product of the neurotransmitters CGRP and SP. CGRP is a potent vasodilator and helps to transmit pain signals and produce needed physiologic inflammation following assault or injury. CGRP has also been shown to increase osteoblast proliferation and activity while decreasing osteoclast maturation. These activities function to build bone in association with normal stress and strain. The neurotransmitter SP is a peptide hormone that is often co-released with CGRP in response to bone stimuli. Similar to CGRP, SP results in local inflammation and vasodilation; however, the end results of this signal are to increase osteoclastogenesis.[11] Current evidence has not yet isolated, and the exact role of SP in bone metabolism and further investigation is required.

CHARCOT NEUROARTHROPATHY

Charcot neuro-osteoarthropathy (CNA) is identified as a rare, yet destructive complication of peripheral neuropathy, which involves marked destruction of bone and joints of the lower extremity. Although not exclusively seen in diabetics, CNA will form in 0.1% to 2.5% of this population, but has been reported in up to 13% of diabetics seen in specialty foot and ankle clinics.[12–14]

Historically, Charcot bone turnover was an anatomic feature identified only through physical and x-ray examination. At the time of its first recording, neuroarthropathy was assumed to have resulted from increased bone perfusion via sympathetic denervation resulting in bone resorption. Charcot was early to identify that the innervation of the bone aided in the nutritional content and metabolism of the local environment. He postulated that disruption of local growth factors led to the ultimate dissolution of the bone,[15] thus giving way to the eventual neurotrophic theory. Predictably, this theory was quickly opposed by the work of Virchow and Volkmann who postulated that sensorial loss allowed for unremitting trauma to the feet and eventual structural damage, also known as the neuro traumatic theory. This theory was also quickly challenged by the work of Corbin and Hinsey,[16] whose denervation studies never produced a single case of neuroarthropathy. It would be another 120 years before any study would use biomarkers to explain the bone pathology of the Charcot foot and ankle. At the time of its initial observation, syphilis was the most common cause of CNA; this etiology has since been replaced by diabetic peripheral neuropathy. This historic observation in the syphilic population is not always easily reconciled with our current models and pathways of pathogenesis. In the last two decades, great awareness of bone turnover in both normal and pathologic models has been identified. Several explanations for pathogenesis have been described; however, a single common pathway has yet to be elucidated. Bone metabolism studies in this population are often descriptive in nature and rarely link markers of bone turnover to causation.

PRO-INFLAMMATORY STATE

Inflammation is an essential stage of bone healing, which involves cytokine activation of osteogenic cells. However, a heightened inflammatory state is potentially pathologic. In the diabetic, and more specifically, the Charcot diabetic population, the prolonged exposure to glycemic dysregulation produces an acute-phase release of cytokines.[17] A pro-inflammatory state is caused by the accumulation of AGE crosslinks, suppression of phosphatidylinositol-3 kinase, and increased protein kinase C activity. In a study by Baumhauer and colleagues,[17] 20 Charcot bone specimens were examined for their histologic and immune reactivity. In these specimens, there was a disproportionate increase in the number of osteoclasts as opposed to osteoblasts. This mismatch suggests a lytic phase of bone change. In addition, they noted increased osteoclastic activity when exposed to the pro-inflammatory cytokines tumor necrosis factor-alpha (TNF-α), interleukin-1b (IL-1b), and interleukin-6 (IL-6). This study correlated elevated cytokine production to increased osteoclast activation in CNA.

Charcot patients were shown to overproduce pro-inflammatory cytokines (TNF-α, IL-1b, and IL-6) and reduce the secretion of the anti-inflammatory cytokines interleukin-4 and interleukin-10 (IL-10).[18] The mismatch between cytokine markers produces a prolonged inflammatory response, which favors osteolysis. Interestingly, in the same study, monocytes taken from these samples showed a resistance to apoptosis allowing for the persistence of osteoclast activity. This study addressed the role those immune-responsive monocytes play in the pathogenesis of Charcot foot. Despite the close association that Charcot pathogenesis shares with inflammation, we have yet to identify a threshold for cytokine activity and the appearance of Charcot foot.

BONE MINERAL DENSITY/CELLULAR CHARACTERISTIC

Bone mineral density (BMD) is a measurement used to assess the mineral content per volume of bone using ultrasound technology. Type II diabetics have historically acknowledged a paradoxic increase in BMD despite an increased risk of fracture. This suggests that BMD may not be an adequate predictor of bone quality. Despite this, several reports have used BMD in the characterization of Charcot bone quality. La Fontaine and colleagues[19] compared quantitative ultrasound of the calcaneus between CNA, diabetics, and healthy controls. In addition, they compared central BMD and peripheral calcaneal stiffness in the same population. This team reported an approximately 36% reduction in calcaneal stiffness in the Charcot population despite nearly comparable central BMD. The authors went on to suggest that enhanced osteoclastogenesis is a local finding and not associated with central osteoporosis. In this same study, samples of bone were taken to reveal a disorganized trabecular pattern that was infiltrated with inflammatory myxoid tissue. The authors identified a tissue that was woven and immature with osteoid-like trabeculations and increased Howship's Lacunae, likely lacking the ability to ossify (**Fig. 1**).

A study performed by Herbst and colleagues[20] associated BMD with their observed subtypes of Charcot foot. In this study, 55 patients were organized into three subtypes: fracture pattern, dislocation pattern, and combined. They recognized that

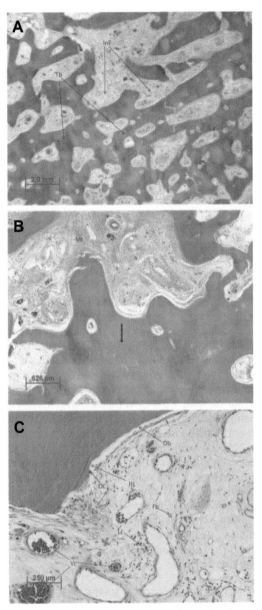

Fig. 1. (*A*) Hematoxylin and eosin stain (1.25x magnification) of CN bone showing thin osteoid-like trabeculae surrounding inflammatory infiltrate (InF). (*B*) Hematoxylin and eosin stain (4x magnification) showing myxoid tissue within InF. Aloes, immature, structurally disorganized bone seen (*black arrow*). (*C*) Hematoxylin and eosin stain (10x magnification) showing a marked increase of osteoclastic activity evidenced by presence of Howship's lacunae and osteoclast, followed by line of osteoblasts. Note: InF dominated by lymphocytes, eosinophils, spindle fibroblasts and significant vascular congestion. (*From* La Fontaine J, Shibuya N, Sampson HW, Valderrama P. Trabecular quality and cellular characteristics of normal, diabetic, and Charcot bone. J Foot Ankle Surg. 2011 Nov-Dec;50(6):648-53. https://doi.org/10.1053/j.jfas.2011.05.005. Epub 2011 Jun 25. PMID: 21705241.)

patients with diminished bone density were at a higher likelihood to develop fracture pattern as opposed to dislocation (**Fig. 2**). In addition, a correlation between anatomic location and subtype was reported. One of the most interesting findings of this study was the recognition of a Charcot subtype, which is without bone dissolution.

The dislocation Charcot subtype has become of increased interest. Several studies have attempted to characterize this subtype.[21,22] A study performed by the investigator correlated fracture pattern to peripheral bone density and level of bone turnover. Evidence from this study identified an increase in bone turnover within the fracture pattern as opposed to dislocation ($P = .05$).[22] In addition, peripheral BMD appeared lower in the fracture pattern as opposed to dislocation ($P < .0001$). Results from this study suggest that there is a subtype of Charcot pathology, which is preserved from heightened bone metabolism and instead results from ligamentous failure.

THE CHARCOT JOINT

Charcot foot pathogenic models are primarily relegated to the description of bone turnover. Few studies have focused on the ligamentous and synovial changes that occur during the collapse. Grant and colleagues[23] evaluated Charcot Achilles tendon samples using electron microscopy (**Fig. 3**). Results from this tendon identified enhanced nonenzymatic collagen cross-linking (AGE) and a mechanic alteration to the Young's modulus of elasticity.[24] These studies support the notion that joint capsules are altered mechanically by the accumulation of AGE.

The synovium lines the inner surface of joints and functions to produce the fluid that nourishes the cartilaginous surface. Along the intimal lining of the capsule are the fibroblast-like synoviocytes (FLSs) that have been associated with other inflammatory disease states (rheumatoid arthritis). When stimulated by inflammatory cytokines, FLS secretes metalloproteinase, which degrades the joint space. Molligan and colleagues[25] took synovial samples from CNA patients and healthy controls to identify the variations in histologic characteristics. Charcot synovium was found to have reduced innervation and marked inflammation. FLSs were cultured from these samples and exposed to TNF-α, which increase their expression of IL-6 and receptor activator of nuclear factor kappa-b ligand (RANKL), and degraded the proteoglycans when cocultured with cartilage.[26] This study identifies that FLS may play an important role in the joint space degradation during the Charcot process. Saloky and colleagues[27] compared fibrillar cartilage density and orientation in synovial tissue of neuropathic patients with and without CNA. The samples of CNA synovium showed a significant reduction in volume fraction, collagen density, and orientation index ($P > .0001$). The qualitative and quantitative difference in Charcot collagen may preclude the joint to eventual collapse.

RECEPTOR ACTIVATOR OF NUCLEAR FACTOR KAPPA-B LIGAND/OSTEOPROTEGRIN SIGNALING

One of the central processes of normal bone metabolism is the receptor activator of nuclear factor kappa-b (RANK), RANKL/osteoprotegrin (OPG) pathway. This pathway has been used to identify pathologic osteolysis in several disease states including rheumatoid arthritis, osteoarthritis, periodontal disease, and peri-prosthetic failure. Macrophage maturation, fusion, and differentiation occur when the RANK ligand binds to its receptor (RANK). This process activates the osteoclast to breakdown bone. The decoy molecule OPG that is produced by osteoblasts and stromal cells then inhibits this process in a classic feedback mechanism (**Fig. 4**). Other cytokines that have been identified that affect this process include TNF-α, IL-10, IL-1, and IL-6. Several

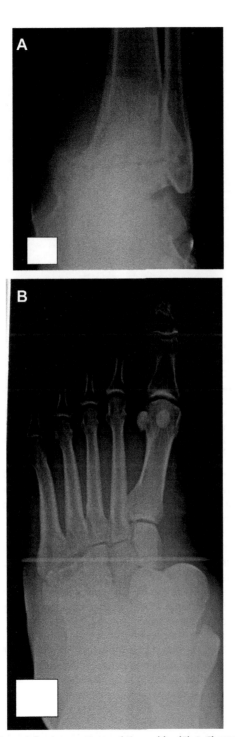

Fig. 2. (*A*) Showing Charcot fracture pattern of the ankle. (*B*) A Charcot dislocation pattern located at the talonavicular joint.

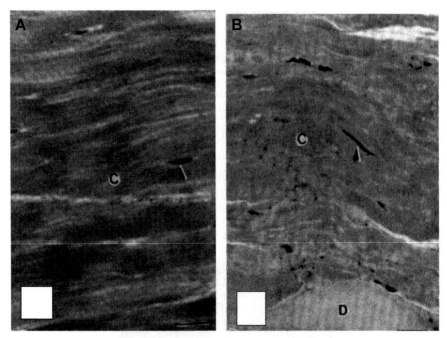

Fig. 3. (*A*) Normal tendon. Aligned and parallel collagen fibrils with no extensive foci of fibrillar disruption. (*B*) Charcot Achilles tendon. Disruption of collagen fibrils with irregular appearance and evidence of cross-linking. (*C*) Compares the structure of collagen between dibetic speciment and controls. (*D*) Represents myxoid degenerative tissue seen in diseased tendon. (*From* Grant WP, Foreman EJ, Wilson AS, Jacobus DA, Kukla RM. Evaluation of Young's modulus in Achilles tendons with diabetic neuroarthropathy. J Am Podiatr Med Assoc. 2005 May-Jun;95(3):242-6. https://doi.org/10.7547/0950242. PMID: 15901810.)

processes seen in diabetics affect the RANKL/OPG pathway. Osteoclast cultures in Charcot patients show more aggressive and mature osteoclasts, which have been abnormally primed for bone breakdown.[28] In addition, they found that activated osteoclasts have insensitivity toward OPG.[18,29] Insensitivity toward the normal negative feedback mechanism suggests that osteoclast activation seen in the Charcot population is likely dually controlled by a RANKL/OPG dependent and independent pathway.

Factors that affect the RANKL/OPG pathway are numerous and often are a byproduct of uncontrolled diabetes mellitus. Hyperglycemia is a known cause of advanced glycated end products and reactive oxygen species, which are powerful inducers of cytokine activation.[30] Pro-inflammatory states are thought to augment the expression of RANKL, leading to osteolysis and increased bone fragility.[31] Interestingly, this pro-inflammatory state is not identified systemically and often the osteolytic destruction is only noted locally.[32] This is thought to represent an immune histologic protection imparted by the body during a biologically damaging process.

NEUROPEPTIDES

The association of Charcot bone metabolism and a CNS abnormality has long been observed but only recently described. Sensorial peripheral neuropathy has been associated with the appearance of elevated markers of IL-1, IL-6, and TNF-α. A potential explanation for this elevation is a mechanically induced microtrauma that causes local

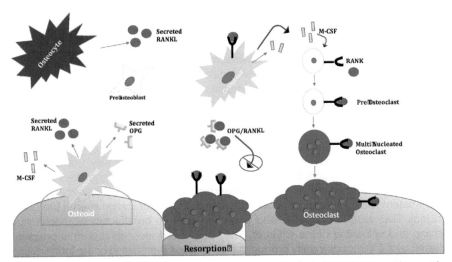

Fig. 4. Intracellular signaling of osteoclast maturation through OPG/RANKL pathway. The mature osteoblast secretes RANKL, OPG, and colony-stimulating factor. RANKL binds to his receptor on the pre-osteoclast to aid in osteoclast maturation. The decoy molecule OPG is used to reduce osteoclast maturation and bind the secreted RANKL.

injury to the bone resulting in inflammatory induced osteolysis. This is a rather simplistic explanation and likely does not represent the full pathogenesis. More recently, this activity is thought to be mediated through peptides that are synthesized by sensory nerves at the end terminus of bones. Similarly, peripheral neuropathy has been associated with CGRP stimulation of osteoclastic activity.[9,33] CGRP is a neuropeptide that is found in the circulatory and digestive systems and aids in the growth of stem cells. The release of the neuropeptides CGRP and SP appears to be non-synaptic and arise from the C fiber and unmylelinated A fiber nerves. CGRP has shown direct regulative control over osteoblasts. In addition, it activates cytokine and growth factor production and synthesis of collagen. CGRP also has anti-inflammatory activity, working to reduce cytokine synthesis. Reduction in the amount of circulating CGRP has been observed in diabetic patients with neuroarthropathy, which may explain the deregulation of their pro-inflammatory state. Moreover, CGRP is a direct inhibitor of osteoclast motility, recruitment, and differentiation. It is, therefore, the postulation that without CGRP inhibition, osteoclasts are recruited in a breakaway feedback loop.[30]

Nitric oxide (NO) is a synaptic neurotransmitter, which plays an important role in numerous regulatory and cell survival mechanisms. NO is a free radical gas that is a secondary messenger in the induction of apoptosis of pre-osteoclasts, signaling cell death. Endothelial nitric oxide synthase, an isoenzyme that regulates NO production, was measured in the Charcot population and found to be significantly reduced as compared with diabetic patients with and without peripheral neuropathy $(P = .008)$.[30] This further catalogs the disruption of osteoclast cell fate and proliferation seen in the Charcot population.

WNT/β-CATENIN SIGNALING PATHWAY

The Wnt signaling pathway, active in both bone and vascular maturation, regulates many essential cellular requirements such as cell polarity, cell fate/maturation, cell migration, formation of cellular axis, and embryonic development. The progression of bone healing is a recapitulation of early embryonic development and uses the same process and pathways.[34,35] Thus, much of what we know regarding bone healing has been borrowed from embryonic development research. There is a large accumulation of data, which identifies the Wnt-β-catenin as a primarily anabolic pathway. Cannonical Wnt signaling results in the translocation of beta-catenin across the nuclear membrane. This translocation allows for the activation of transcription factors, which activate genes responsible for cellular development. Involved in this pathway is the signal protein sclerostin, a protein that is produced by osteocytes to inhibit bone formation as a response to the reduction in mechanical loading. High levels of sclerostin activate osteocytes and result in low bone mass. Conversely, the signal protein Dickkopf-1 (Dkk-1) acts as an antagonist to the Wnt pathway and plays a crucial role in bone formation. Folestad and colleagues[36] identified a potential role that the Wnt/β-catenin pathway is responsible for the anabolic manifestation seen in the Charcot foot. They found both Dkk-1 and sclerostin seem to be affected by mechanical loading and unloading of the Charcot. They postulated that the abnormal pressure created by a Charcot deformity produces a continuous remodeling of the foot, limiting the ability for the bone to mature.

COLLAGEN CROSS-LINKING AND ADVANCED GLYCATION END PRODUCTS/RECEPTOR FOR ADVANCED GLYCATION END PRODUCTS

Nonenzymatic glycation is a process that allows glucose to attach to lipids and proteins without the use of an enzymatic intermediary. Advanced glycated end products have been identified in various tissues throughout the body and have been implicated in numerous disease states (cardiovascular disease, end-stage renal disease, and neuropathy).[37,38] AGEs are often found in tissues with a lower rate of turnover (ie, cortical bone). Enzymatic collagen cross-linking is important to the tensile strength of bone; however, the accumulation of nonenzymatic cross-linking (AGE) has been associated with poor mineralization because of inhibition of osteoblast maturation and impairment of osteoblastic adhesion to bone surfaces. In addition, pathologic cross-linking causes rigidity of collagen fibers and reduction in fatigue resistance.[24] The receptor for advanced glycation end products (RAGEs) is a member of the immunoglobulin superfamily of cell surface molecules. RAGE has multiple ligand receptors and works as a mediator to inflammatory and immune responses. These receptors are found on pro-inflammatory cells such as neutrophils, monocytes, macrophages, and T and B lymphocytes. The binding of AGE to its receptor activates the production of more receptors, ultimately perpetuating inflammation. RAGE production and function are controlled through ligand binding and of the RAGE isoform soluble RAGE (sRAGE). Soluble RAGE can bind to pro-inflammatory ligands, thus blocking the binding of RAGE and inhibiting the pro-inflammatory state. In this way, sRAGE is a protective molecule, which favors anti-inflammatory effects. In a study by Witzke and colleagues,[39] Charcot patients had an 86% reduction in circulating sRAGE as compared with healthy controls. Furthermore, there was a positive correlation between reduction in calcaneal stiffness and circulating sRAGE ($P < .001$). These findings taken together suggest that Charcot patient's loss of sRAGE defense may increase bone turnover related to a RANK independent pathway.

CHARCOT BONE THERAPEUTICS OPTIONS

Medicinal treatment of the Charcot foot and ankle has undergone a great deal of change in the last 20 years. Given the greater understanding of the pathophysiology of this condition, advancements in oral therapies have become a topic of interest. Bisphosphonates are a class of drugs that slow or prevent the resorption of bone by osteoclasts. There is further evidence to suggest that these drugs may also inhibit the proliferation of osteoblasts, leading to the potential negative consequence of fatigue fracture. The bisphosphonate pamidronate functions by irreversibly binding to hydroxyapatite and preventing the access of osteoclast precursor cells to the bone matrix. Using this drug, Jude and colleagues[40] followed 39 active phase Charcot patients in a double-blind placebo-controlled trial to identify the 1-year efficacy of bisphosphonates. Patients in this trial who received a single dose of 90-mg pamidronate experienced a significant reduction in bone turnover ($P = .01$) and resolution of inflammation ($P < .001$) as compared with placebo. In a similar study, Pitocco and colleagues[41] used 70 mg alendronate in 11 blinded and randomized patients for comparison to nine controls. They found a statistical significance in improvement in bone density ($P < .05$), reduction in pain ($P < .05$), and resolution of inflammation ($P < .05$). No negative side effects were noted in the test population, and the authors identified overall improvement in markers of bone resorption. In a contradictory study, Pakarinen and colleagues[42] followed 39 active Charcot patients and randomized half into a Zoledronic acid treatment group. They compared the resolution of symptoms and return to weight bearing. This study identified a prolonged immobilization in the treatment group as compared with controls ($P = .02$). The authors went on to suggest that the use of bisphosphonates might in fact prolong the active phase of the disease. This team advocated instead for further investigation into medications that target the RANKL/OPG pathway or its intermediaries (TNF-α, NF-kB).

Intranasal calcitonin has been studied in the Charcot population as a potential inhibitor of the RANKL/OPG system, thus preventing osteoclastic bone destruction. In addition, intranasal calcitonin does not seem to interfere with osteoblast activity, diminishing the risk of fatigue fracture. As an added advantage, calcitonin is safe to use in renal insufficiency, allowing a wider population of diabetics to be treated. Bem and colleagues[43] followed 32 CNA patients and divided them into two treatment groups: 200 IU daily intranasal calcitonin and calcium supplementation. A significant difference was seen in clinical symptoms ($P < .01$) and markers of bone turnover ($P < .05$). The authors reported an improved safety profile and a more inclusive patient population.

NF-kB antibody (denosumab) has been used to treat osteoporosis-related fracture and several bone-related tumors and was identified as a possible treatment of acute-phase CNA. NF-kB is a known arbitrator to osteoclastogenesis and thus is enhanced in bone lytic states. Denosumab has been branded as a safe medication with a known adverse effect of hypocalcemia; therefore, calcium supplementation and testing are required in follow-up. In a study by Busch-Westbroek and colleagues, 11 active Charcot patients were treated with a single dose of 60 mg denosumab sub-Q and compared with historic controls.[44] The treatment group was noted to have a significant reduction in fracture resolution ($P < .01$) and less malalignment ($P < .01$) than the control group. Similar studies have since echoed these findings; however, most all continue to show small population sizes with relatively little inference made to the larger population.

SUMMARY

Charcot bone metabolism went largely unexplored for more than 120 years. With a renewed clinical focus, a drastic change to the once barren landscape has occurred in just the past two decades. It is clear that no single metabolic pathway explains all

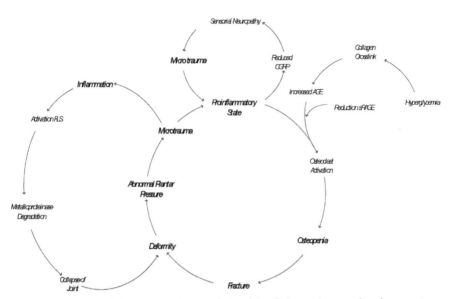

Fig. 5. A schematic of the proposed interrelationship of the pathways of pathogenesis.

of the varied findings of the Charcot foot and ankle. The progression of this disorder is likely exaggerated through a pro-inflammatory state and advanced autonomic peripheral neuropathy, which is amplified through reduction in sRAGE, a collection of AGEs and accumulation of oxidative stress. Once that patient has reached an unknown threshold of cytokine activation, monoclonal cells are signaled for differentiation and primed for continuous osteolysis. Osteoclasts under the control of RANKL dependent and independent signaling anabolize the bone, whereas osteoblast cells are unable to differentiate and undergo cellular apoptosis. In addition, advanced autonomic peripheral neuropathy reduces the level of CGRP at the n-terminus of bone, diminishing the amount of anti-inflammatory effects released at the trophic sites. The disordered cross-linking of collagen leads to the weakening of joint capsules and eventual dislocation. Again, the exaggerated inflammatory state activates FLS cells to release metalloproteinase, which destroys cartilage and subchondral bone. Once the foot has collapsed, the abnormal plantar pressure caused by a rocker bottom deformity limits the ability for a Wnt pathway to mature the bone. The end result is bone that is woven and lacks the appropriate quality to resist compression and shear forces (**Fig. 5**).

An individual with this combination of nerve and AGE accumulation will always be at risk for reactivation of the cytokine storm, which precipitates active bone destruction. Despite a greater understanding of the metabolic abnormality of the Charcot foot, the efforts to establish a single, common pathway with a known threshold of activation are still desired. The therapeutic trial is still in its infancy and with greater understanding of metabolic pathways, a better solution may be soon discovered.

REFERENCES

1. Datta HK, Ng WF, Walker JA, et al. The cell biology of bone metabolism. J Clin Pathol 2008;61(5):577–87.

2. Dimar JR, Lane JM, Lehman RA Jr, et al. The basics of bone physiology, healing, and osteoporosis. Instr Course Lect 2021;70:527–36.

3. Hart NH, Newton RU, Tan J, et al. Biological basis of bone strength: anatomy, physiology and measurement. J Musculoskelet Neuronal Interact 2020;20(3): 347–71.
4. Rowe P, Koller A, Sharma S. Physiology, bone remodeling. Treasure Island (FL): StatPearls; 2021.
5. Zhang K, Liu X, Wang L, et al. The mechanosensory and mechanotransductive processes mediated by ion channels and the impact on bone metabolism: a systematic review. Arch Biochem Biophys 2021;711:109020.
6. Saito M, Marumo K. [Roles of collagen enzymatic and advanced glycation end products associated crosslinking as a determinant of bone quality]. Nihon Rinsho 2011;69(7):1189–97.
7. Chenu C. Role of innervation in the control of bone remodeling. J Musculoskelet Neuronal Interact 2004;4(2):132–4.
8. Togari A. Adrenergic regulation of bone metabolism: possible involvement of sympathetic innervation of osteoblastic and osteoclastic cells. Microsc Res Tech 2002;58(2):77–84.
9. Chen J, Ma G, Liu W, et al. The influence of the sensory neurotransmitter calcitonin gene-related peptide on bone marrow mesenchymal stem cells from ovariectomized rats. J Bone Miner Metab 2017;35(5):473–84.
10. Skerry TM. Neurotransmitter functions in bone remodeling. J Musculoskelet Neuronal Interact 2002;2(3):281.
11. Spencer GJ, Hitchcock IS, Genever PG. Emerging neuroskeletal signalling pathways: a review. FEBS Lett 2004;559(1–3):6–12.
12. Papa J, Myerson M, Girard P. Salvage, with arthrodesis, in intractable diabetic neuropathic arthropathy of the foot and ankle. J Bone Joint Surg Am 1993; 75(7):1056–66.
13. Sinha S, Munichoodappa CS, Kozak GP. Neuro-arthropathy (Charcot joints) in diabetes mellitus (clinical study of 101 cases). Medicine (Baltimore) 1972; 51(3):191–210.
14. Armstrong DG, Todd WF, Lavery LA, et al. The natural history of acute Charcot's arthropathy in a diabetic foot specialty clinic. Diabet Med 1997;14(5):357–63.
15. Charcot JM. Sur quelquesarthropathiesqui paraissent dependre d'une lesion du cerveauou de la mouelle 'espiniere. Arch Physiol Norm Pathol 1968;1:161–78.
16. Corbin, Kendall B, Joseph CHinsey. Influence of the nervous system on bone and joints. The Anatomical Record 1939;75(3):307–17.
17. Baumhauer JF, O'Keefe RJ, Schon LC, et al. Cytokine-induced osteoclastic bone resorption in charcot arthropathy: an immunohistochemical study. Foot Ankle Int 2006;27(10):797–800.
18. Uccioli L, Sinistro A, Almerighi C, et al. Proinflammatory modulation of the surface and cytokine phenotype of monocytes in patients with acute Charcot foot. Diabetes Care 2010;33(2):350–5.
19. La Fontaine J, Shibuya N, Sampson HW, et al. Trabecular quality and cellular characteristics of normal, diabetic, and charcot bone. J Foot Ankle Surg 2011; 50(6):648–53.
20. Herbst SA, Jones KB, Saltzman CL. Pattern of diabetic neuropathic arthropathy associated with the peripheral bone mineral density. J Bone Joint Surg Br 2004;86(3):378–83.
21. Cates, Nicole. Risk Factors and Outcomes After Surgical Reconstruction of Charcot Neuroarthropathy in Fracture Versus Dislocation Patterns. The Journal of Foot and Ankle Surgery 2022;61(2):264–71.

22. Grant L, Yoho R, Halaharvi C, et al. Charcot collapse: does collapse pattern dictate osseous metabolism? Foot Ankle Spec 2017;10(5):428–34.

23. Grant WP, Sullivan R, Sonenshine DE, et al. Electron microscopic investigation of the effects of diabetes mellitus on the Achilles tendon. J Foot Ankle Surg 1997; 36(4):272–8 [discussion: 330].

24. Grant WP, Foreman EJ, Wilson AS, et al. Evaluation of Young's modulus in Achilles tendons with diabetic neuroarthropathy. J Am Podiatr Med Assoc 2005;95(3): 242–6.

25. Molligan J, Barr C, Mitchell R, et al. Pathological role of fibroblast-like synovio-cytes in charcot neuroarthropathy. J Orthop Res 2016;34(2):224–30.

26. Mitchell R, Molligan J, Rooney S, et al. Functionally compromised synovium-derived mesenchymal stem cells in Charcot neuroarthropathy. Exp Mol Pathol 2018;104(1):82–8.

27. Kairlin Saloky CA, Walley K, Aynardi M. Thomas abraham quantitative assess-ments of remodeling of fibrillar collagens in charcot neuroarthropathy. Orthopae-dic Jounral Harv Med Sch 2020;21:7–13.

28. Mabilleau G, Petrova N, Edmonds ME, et al. Number of circulating CD14-positive cells and the serum levels of TNF-alpha are raised in acute charcot foot. Diabetes Care 2011;34(3):e33.

29. Mangan DF, Welch GR, Wahl SM. Lipopolysaccharide, tumor necrosis factor-alpha, and IL-1 beta prevent programmed cell death (apoptosis) in human pe-ripheral blood monocytes. J Immunol 1991;146(5):1541–6.

30. La Fontaine J, Harkless LB, Sylvia VL, et al. Levels of endothelial nitric oxide syn-thase and calcitonin gene-related peptide in the Charcot foot: a pilot study. J Foot Ankle Surg 2008;47(5):424–9.

31. Jeffcoate W, Game F, Cavanagh PR. The role proinflammatory cytokines in the cuase of neurpathic osteoarthropathy in diabetes. Lancet 2005;366:2058–61.

32. Ndip A, Williams A, Jude EB, et al. The RANKL/RANK/OPG signaling pathway mediates medial arterial calcification in diabetic Charcot neuroarthropathy. Dia-betes 2011;60(8):2187–96.

33. Akopian A, Demulder A, Ouriaghli F, et al. Effects of CGRP on human osteoclast-like cell formation: a possible connection with the bone loss in neurological disor-ders? Peptides 2000;21(4):559–64.

34. Lojk J, Marc J. Roles of non-canonical Wnt signalling pathways in bone biology. Int J Mol Sci 2021;22(19):10840.

35. Schupbach D, Comeau-Gauthier M, Harvey E, et al. Wnt modulation in bone heal-ing. Bone 2020;138:115491.

36. Folestad A, Alund M, Asteberg S, et al. Role of Wnt/beta-catenin and RANKL/ OPG in bone healing of diabetic Charcot arthropathy patients. Acta Orthop 2015;86(4):415–25.

37. Yamagishi SI. Role of advanced glycation endproduct (AGE)-Receptor for advanced glycation endproduct (RAGE) Axis in cardiovascular disease and its therapeutic intervention. Circ J 2019;83(9):1822–8.

38. Smit AJ, Gerrits EG. Skin autofluorescence as a measure of advanced glycation endproduct deposition: a novel risk marker in chronic kidney disease. Curr Opin Nephrol Hypertens 2010;19(6):527–33.

39. Witzke KA, Vinik AI, Grant LM, et al. Loss of RAGE defense: a cause of Charcot neuroarthropathy? Diabetes Care 2011;34(7):1617–21.

40. Jude EB, Selby PL, Burgess J, et al. Bisphosphonates in the treatment of Charcot neuroarthropathy: a double-blind randomised controlled trial. Diabetologia 2001; 44(11):2032–7.

41. Pitocco D, Ruotolo V, Caputo S, et al. Six-month treatment with alendronate in acute Charcot neuroarthropathy: a randomized controlled trial. Diabetes Care 2005;28(5):1214–5.
42. Pakarinen TK, Laine HJ, Maenpaa H, et al. Effect of immobilization, off-loading and zoledronic acid on bone mineral density in patients with acute Charcot neuroarthropathy: a prospective randomized trial. Foot Ankle Surg 2013;19(2):121–4.
43. Bem R, Jirkovska A, Fejfarova V, et al. Intranasal calcitonin in the treatment of acute Charcot neuroosteoarthropathy: a randomized controlled trial. Diabetes Care 2006;29(6):1392–4.
44. Busch-Westbroek TE, Delpeut K, Balm R, et al. Effect of single dose of RANKL antibody treatment on acute charcot neuro-osteoarthropathy of the foot. Diabetes Care 2018;41(3):e21–2.

Management of the Charcot Foot and Ankle
Nonreconstructive Surgery

Shirley Chen, DPM, John D. Miller, DPM, John S. Steinberg, DPM*

KEYWORDS

- Nonreconstructive surgery • Diabetic foot deformity • Amputation • Charcot surgery
- charcot arthropathy

KEY POINTS

- charcot arthropathy is a devastating condition.
- Soft tissue balancing and tendon transfers can be used in correction of Charcot deformity.
- Any Charcot patient undergoing surgery should have thorough preoperative work-up including vascular and metabolic studies.
- Nonsalvageable limbs should be considered for early amputation.

INTRODUCTION

The modern understanding and surgical management of charcot arthropathy and its sequelae has undergone a renaissance in the new millennium. A combination of advances in surgical instrumentation and the evolution of evidence and outcomes based-practice have led to significant improvements in the long-term functional outcomes of patients with Charcot arthropathy and in reducing long-term major amputation rates. The application of these practices has produced more efficient utilization of patient-specific treatments and a better appreciation of this complex pathologic condition. Despite these advancements, Charcot arthropathy imparts a significant burden on the health-care system at large and on the wellbeing of those patients suffering from this devastating condition. In this article, we will focus on modern techniques for nonreconstructive surgical management of patients with charcot arthropathy who have failed conservative management.

Department of Plastic Surgery, Georgetown University School of Medicine, MedStar Washington Hospital Center Podiatric Surgery Residency, Center for Wound Healing, MedStar Georgetown University Hospital, 3800 Reservoir Road Northwest, Bles Building 1st Floor, Washington, DC 20007, USA
* Corresponding author.
E-mail address: john.steinberg@medstar.net

Clin Podiatr Med Surg 39 (2022) 559–570
https://doi.org/10.1016/j.cpm.2022.05.003   **podiatric.theclinics.com**
0891-8422/22/© 2022 Elsevier Inc. All rights reserved.

Initial Management

Charcot arthropathy is a progressive and devastating condition that involves both a loss of sensory nerve function combined with dynamic vascular changes that leads to bone and joint deformation and fragmentation. If not diagnosed and treated early and aggressively, the consequences from collapsed joints (**Fig. 1**), instability, and deformity subject the foot to bony prominences, leading to ulceration and potential infection.[1] Prophylactic measures at the original diagnosis include offloading the foot to prevent further collapse and break down through total contact casting, as well as bracing and accommodation of any bony prominences that may have developed with an ankle foot orthoses or Charcot Restraint Orthotic Walker.[2] This is imperative during the acute stages of Charcot through coalescent and remodeling stages to ensure the foot is offloaded until there is some stability restored in the foot.

If an ulcer does develop before or despite offloading and bracing, diligent wound care, offloading, and surgical debridement as indicated are critical to infection management and amputation prevention. Ulcers that are acute and free of infection can be treated with local debridement to bleeding tissue using any combination of instruments in the clinic setting including curettes, blades, and rongeurs or scissors. Chronic ulcers that have remained recalcitrant in healing, larger sized wounds in precarious or high-pressure locations, or those with concomitant soft tissue or bone infection may require more aggressive surgical debridement in the operating room. Surgical debridement may provide more definitive resection of infected or nonviable tissue and may also allow for surgical excision and primary wound closure.[3] Other techniques such as local muscle or skin flaps, free tissue flaps, split thickness or full thickness skin grafting, and biologics may be used to facilitate closure of the wound and coverage over the bone depending on the tissue, osseous geography, and surgeon skill set available.[4]

A Candidate for Reconstructive or Nonreconstructive Surgery?

Ideally every collapsed or deformed Charcot foot could be surgically restored into a biomechanically sound and ambulatory segment. However, oftentimes multiple patient factors prevent patients from being optimal surgical candidates for the level of reconstruction required. This largely depends on the patient's ability to undergo a major reconstructive 3 to 5 hour surgery under general anesthesia and their healing potentials for both large soft tissue incisions and dissections, and ability to heal bones that are fused to prevent recollapse and hardware failure.[5,6]

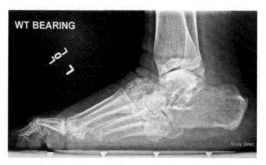

Fig. 1. Lateral weight-bearing radiograph demonstrating disruption of normal midfoot and midfoot alignment secondary to charcot arthropathy, now consolidated. Continued midfoot collapse often leads to plantar midfoot ulceration requiring surgical intervention.

Thorough preoperative evaluation must be performed for all patients to determine whether they are best suited for conservative therapy, nonreconstructive, or reconstructive surgery. Laboratory testing necessary for ruling out underlying osteomyelitis before reconstructive surgery includes complete blood cell count with differential, basic metabolic panel, C-reactive protein, and erythrocyte sedimentation rate. Additionally, suspicion for osteomyelitis may also be evaluated using advanced imaging such as magnetic resonance imaging or cell-labeled bone scans, bone biopsies with culture and/or pathologic condition results, and associated clinical findings.[7] If a reasonable concern for infection remains, reconstruction of the foot with hardware should be postponed until infection can either be eliminated via parenteral antibiotics, aggressive debridement, or by segmental amputation when indicated.[8]

Central to determining a patient's candidacy for surgical reconstruction is their level of vascular inflow to target operative areas. Determining and maximizing peripheral vascular patency is imperative to any surgical procedure, and it is particularly important for a major reconstructive surgery to avoid wound healing complications. Doppler ultrasound tests, ankle brachial index (ABI)'s/pulse volume recording (PVR)'s and other noninvasive studies are critical for detecting and improving surgical outcomes in CNA patients.[9] Proper vascular studies or angiography will guide surgical planning whether a planned partial foot amputation, tendon transfer, or a reconstruction can be amenable to healing based on incision placement of the indicated procedure.[10,11]

Another important consideration is a patient's comorbidities with uncontrolled diabetes, morbid obesity, localized osteopenia, deficiency of endogenous growth factors, or other immunocompromising diseases impairing the ability to heal bone and soft tissue. Strict glycemic control of blood sugars less than 200 mg/dL and an optimized hemoglobin A1C should be implemented before any surgery to optimize healing potential in both reconstructive and nonreconstructive surgeries.[12] Poorly controlled blood glucose levels are associated with elevated rates of postoperative complication and may be independent risk factors for proximal amputation.[13]

Finally, postoperative management and rehabilitation often requires extensive resources and patient diligence, particularly as the extent of surgical extent expands. Therefore, extensive reconstruction of Charcot arthropathy may at times be reserved for patients who have adequate outpatient support and can demonstrate the patient compliance required during extended recovery. Such patients may necessitate several months of strict nonweight-bearing as well as the resources and support system through the recovery period to ensure success in the postoperative period. Oftentimes, environmental and social factors prohibit the patient from the strict postoperative course of a reconstruction and may be suited better with nonreconstructive surgical options we will discuss below.[14]

Ostectomies/Plantar Exostectomies

Charcot arthropathy is a progressive, deforming process in which the normal ligamentous and osseous architecture of the anatomic segment is lost. Patients who fail off-loading and accommodation commonly form a severe rocker-bottom deformity of the midfoot, and develop prominent osseous exostosis, which can form pressure-related ulcerations.[13] Surgical ostectomy or exostectomy at areas of bony prominences may offer a nonconstructive method to remove the offending pressure and allow for ulcerative healing. One of the most important factors for determining whether to perform an ostectomy is stability through the foot. Patients with gross instability in the foot may result in further instability with aggressive removal of bone and recollapse. Ostectomy is reserved for patients in the late stage of charcot arthropathy to ensure complete coalescence and that the process has completed its course and has an accessible apex of deformity to remove.[15]

There are several considerations when planning the approach for surgical resection of offending osseous structures. First, resection may be performed through either a direct or an indirect approach. A direct approach accesses the underlying bone through the apex of deformity and also allows any existing wound to be excised and closed concomitantly. An indirect approach uses a separate incision (typically either on the medial or lateral foot depending on apex of deformity) and allows planing of the osseous prominence without necessitating incision on a plantar weight-bearing surface.[16]

Dissection should be carried down to provide enough exposure to the underlying bone and to free any soft tissue or periosteal attachments. It is however important to avoid unnecessary dissection that may destabilize adjacent bones and joints that can result in a progression of the deformity. Utilization of full thickness flaps may prevent vascular disruption associated with excessive dissection and maintain flap perfusion for closure. Offending bone is then removed with a sagittal saw, large osteotomes, or rongeurs ensuring adequate bone resection to prevent recurrence of the high-pressure area. Care must be taken to avoid overresection, which may lead to instability following surgery.[17]

Considerations for closure may be primary closure if there was initially a closed-soft tissue envelope or there is a wound that can be primarily excised and closed. A delayed primary closure should be considered in cases of soft tissue or bone infection or offloading, vacuum-assisted closure or biologics for wounds that are not able to be primarily closed. A closed suction drain may be considered in patients with a closed soft tissue envelope as exposed cancellous surfaces following ostectomy can result in significant bleeding.

The postoperative course may vary between patients based on the location of the ostectomy and whether the wound or incision was primarily closed. Offloading the patient in a period of nonweight-bearing or partial weight-bearing is required to allow the incision or the wound to completely heal. Complications following an ostectomy surgery include failure of the ulcer to heal, as well as recurrence of an ulcer secondary to continued anatomic collapse.[16]

Limited level 1 or 2 evidence-based medicine studies exist regarding the long-term effectiveness of ostectomies in symptomatic charcot arthropathy. In a review of 27 patients who underwent ostectomies, Catanzariti and colleagues found wounds resolved in 20/27 cases. Notably, the wounds that failed to heal were in patients with grossly unstable feet and when wounds were beneath the lateral column.[16] In their findings, 92% of ulcers under the medial column healed, compared with only 37.5% under the lateral column following a single exostectomy.[16] These findings were similar to Laurinaviciene and colleagues who performed an exostectomy in 20 consecutive patients with charcot arthropathy and a nonhealing plantar ulceration. Despite an eventual healing rate of 90%, the patients experienced 9 return ulcerations, 6 of which were beneath the lateral column and required repeated planing for resolution.[18] This concept is reinforced by Cates and colleagues who noted that the dislocation pattern Charcot has statistically significant higher rates of broken hardware and requires higher rates of revisional exostectomy compared with pure fracture pattern Charcot.[11]

Brodsky and colleagues had noted that 11 out of 12 patients who had ostectomies for their plantar prominences healed their wounds without subsequent breakdown or new exostosis formation.[15] One patient required a repeat exostectomy, followed by a Syme's amputation. The remaining 11 patients healed with no subsequent breakdown during the 25 month follow-up period.[15] Rosenblum noted a 89% overall success rate with 29 of 32 patient maintaining functional limb salvage after lateral column exostectomy with adjuvant procedures of excising and closing the wound, rotational fasciocutaneous flaps, intrinsic muscle flaps, and with incision lateral to the ulcer.[19] Despite lacking level 1 evidence, these collected case series demonstrate a high rate of success and safety when planing predominantly medial midfoot exostosis with ulceration following charcot arthropathy.

Muscle Flaps

Muscle flaps were first introduced by Ger in the 1960s and have gained popularity and utility given their low donor site morbidity and durability to fill a dead space and defects.[20] Common intrinsic muscles used given their location are the flexor digitorum brevis, abductor hallucis, and abductor digiti minimi plantar foot wounds. These muscles are harvested by transection distally and raised to visualize perforating vessels. The most proximal vessels are preserved to ensure viability of the muscle flap and the distal end of the muscle is rotated to contour the void of the ulcer while the donor site is closed primarily. These muscle flaps may be used in conjunction with ostectomies or offloading to provide a versatility to soft tissue coverage as well as vascularity to soft tissue and devitalized bone (**Fig. 2A–C**).[21,22]

Soft Tissue Correction

Although the deforming force in charcot arthropathy is largely osseous in nature, there are soft tissue forces that may contribute to the progression of the deformity.

Equinus correction

Assessing for equinus in patients with Charcot arthropathy is important during surgical planning. An equinus contracture is defined by limited ankle joint range of motion secondary to tightness or shortening of the Achilles tendon.[23] Motor neuropathy in Charcot patients causes a motor imbalance, which leads to a gastrocnemius-soleus and/or an Achilles tendon contracture and equinus deformity.[24] In the presence of peripheral neuropathy, the increased plantarflexion caused by equinus may affect the joint forces and plantar pressures that contribute to the progression of charcot arthropathy. Addressing the posterior compartment and surgically lengthening it to increase ankle joint dorsiflexion may evenly distribute and offload plantar pressures distally in the foot or at the area of Charcot breakdown preventing further osseous and soft tissue breakdown.[25] Hastings demonstrated lengthening the Achilles tendon improves ankle dorsiflexion, decreased peak plantar pressures, and

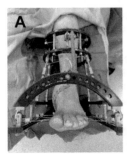
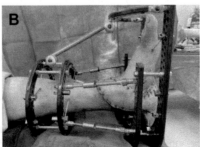
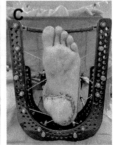

Fig. 2. (*A–C*) A case with significant plantar and medial soft tissue loss requiring free arterial flap and external fixator for offloading. Use of external fixation permits earlier weight-bearing for transfers, which would otherwise be prohibited.

improved overall walking in a diabetic patient.[24] Greenhagen thought a gastrocnemius recession could prevent its development of the Charcot foot by decreasing its causative forces.[26]

Surgical procedures may address specifically lengthening the Achilles tendon through a percutaneous tendo-Achilles lengthening, a gastrocnemius recession, or a complete tenotomy. A percutaneous tendo-Achilles lengthening through the use of a Hoke triple hemisection technique is one of the most popular procedures for lengthening an Achilles tendon given its simplicity.[27] Open lengthening may be performed as well for more severe contractures, which allows for more control over how much tendon is lengthened. There are several procedures described in the literature for gastrocnemius recessions including but not limited to a Vulpius, Strayer, Baker, and Baumann.[24] It is important to be cautious not to over lengthen or iatrogenically rupture the Achilles tendon while performing the procedure, which may lead to an antalgic or calcaneal gait. A calcaneal gait may result in plantar calcaneal ulcerations, which are challenging to heal. Overcorrecting or undercorrecting the equinus deformity can also lead to unstable pressures at other joints causing a Charcot event elsewhere.

Hansen and colleagues have shown and advocate for early lengthening of the Achilles tendon or gastrocnemius recession to minimize the development of Charcot arthropathy.[28] Tiruveedhula performed tendo Achilles lengthening in 33 feet of patients with midfoot Charcot and noted that in 30 out of 33 feet, the disease progression stopped or offloaded preulcerative lesions.[29] In a case report, Holthusen found radiographic improvement in the midfoot arch after Achilles tendon lengthening.[30] Gastrocnemius recessions can be advantageous to tendo Achilles lengthenings because it gives a more controlled soft tissue release, reduces the risk of overlengthening, maintains plantarflexory strength, and reduces the risk of Achilles tendon rupture. Laborde performed gastrocnemius recessions in 21 patients (25 feet) as the primary treatment of midfoot Charcot arthropathy, and 22 of 25 feet went to heal their wounds completely without transfer ulcerations in any of the patients.[31,32] Despite remaining a current standard of care, no level 1 studies exist regarding the efficacy of posterior compartment lengthening in the management of charcot arthropathy deformity with equinus contracture.

Anterior tibialis and posterior tibialis transfers

With the loss of sensation, loss of innervation of motor nerves and muscle function in patients, tendon imbalances occur in the population of Charcot patients particularly after partial foot amputation that result in further anatomic foot deformities (**Fig. 3**A, B).[33] Although there have been many studies on tendo Achilles lengthening procedures as adjuvant procedures for tendon rebalancing, there are fewer published studies on tendon imbalances to correct residual varus deformities such as tibialis anterior and tibialis posterior tendon transfers.

Partial or midfoot amputations such as a transmetatarsal amputation, Lisfranc amputation, or Charcot amputation are typically performed in the setting of acute soft tissue or bone infection to prevent further proximal limb loss. These partial foot amputations however do not address the underlying Charcot deformity and may result in a more varus deformity due to a few factors. The loss of the forefoot eliminates the weight-bearing aspect of the transverse arch of the foot resulting in a forefoot varus. Moreover, the loss of the intrinsic musculature insertions and plantar fascia leads to both instability and loss of the windlass mechanism, which is responsible for raising the longitudinal arch of the foot and subsequent lowering of the medial aspect of the foot.[34]

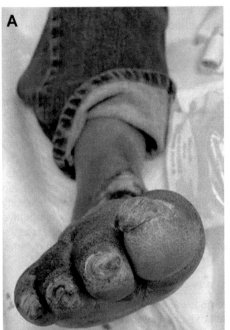 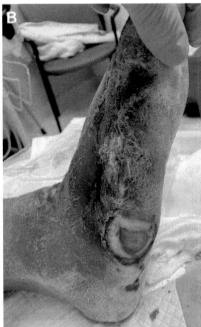

Fig. 3. (*A*) A patient with notable varus deformity following fifth ray resection. Patient is now seen with a wound to the remaining lateral midfoot (*B*), which may benefit from TA or PT tendon transfer to remove supinatory forces. PT, posterior tibial; TA, tibialis anterior.

Patients who have an existing varus deformity before amputation may also develop prominent lateral wounds particularly over the fifth metatarsal base that may require resection of the fifth metatarsal along with the insertion of the peroneus brevis tendon. This in turn results in more advantage of the anterior and posterior tibialis tendons, and a tendon transfer would likely need to be considered to prevent further equinovarus deformity.[35]

The anterior tibial tendon transfer (ATTT) was first described in 1940 for the correction of residual pediatric clubfoot.[36] Since then, the indications for the ATTT have expanded, and ATTT has been used in the diabetic population particularly after partial foot amputation with residual varus deformities. Transfer of the anterior tibial tendon to redistribute the forces prevents further Charcot breakdown in other joints. The tendon transfer involves the complete removal of the tendon at its insertion and subsequently transferring it to the lateral aspect of the foot, generally the lateral cuneiform or cuboid depending on the length of the tendon harvest in a patient with a transmetatarsal or lisfranc amputation or to the talar neck in a Chopart amputation. This transfer can effectively balance the foot by increasing everting forces and decreasing lateral column load and further collapse.[35]

Transfer of the posterior tibial tendon to the dorsal foot was first described by Ober in 1933.[37] Putti discussed transferring the tendon through the interosseous membrane in 1937 but the procedure was popularized by Watkins in 1955.[38] Transfer for this tendon to the dorsum of the foot is mainly indicated for dorsiflexory weakness but is widely used now to aid in eversion in the setting of a varus deformity or peroneal weakness secondary to motor neuropathy.[39] Because this is an out-of-phase transfer, muscle strength must be assessed preoperatively to ensure adequate strength because one grade of strength will be lost after transfer. The posterior tibial tendon is resected in total from its insertion and routed posterior to anterior through the interosseous membrane to be transferred to the dorsal lateral aspect of the foot to balance out the inverters of the foot.

External Fixation

The use of external fixation has gained popularity in the most recent years as a less invasive alternative to complex reconstruction of Charcot arthropathy.[40–42] The advantages of using external fixation are reserved for patients with chronic wounds, osteomyelitis, a poor soft tissue envelope, severe bone loss with osteopenia, morbid obesity or multiple comorbidities not suitable for foot reconstruction with internal fixation. This is a salvage treatment of patients who may otherwise require amputation.[40–42] Circular fixators with either small wire or half pin fixation may be applied when there is an open wound for offloading and stabilization of the deformity (**Fig. 4**). Dalla Paola and colleagues demonstrated external fixation as an alternative to amputation in certain patients following 39 of 45 patients with charcot arthropathy healing their wounds after emergent surgery to drain an acute infection with external fixation after a period of 25.7 weeks.[43]

Nonsalvageable Extremities

Unfortunately, nearly 200,000 patients undergo lower extremity amputation annually in the United States, with nearly 80% the result of ischemia or infection. In cases where charcot arthropathy in a lower extremity has evolved to the extent of nonreconstructable soft tissue (**Fig. 5**) or osseous (**Fig. 6**A, B) structures, lower extremity amputation should be considered. As the 5 year mortality rate following lower extremity

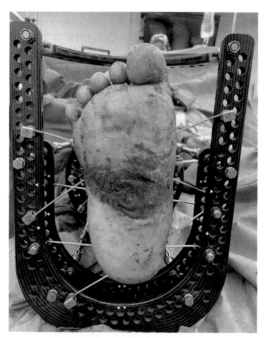

Fig. 4. Case demonstration of plantar excision prominent plantar cuboid bone and primary wound closure with application offloading frame to promote healing.

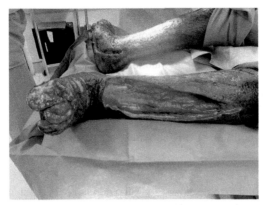

Fig. 5. Below case demonstrates an unfortunate patient with nonreconstructable soft tissue envelope who may benefit from either below or above knee amputation for resolution of lower extremity charcot arthropathy with osteomyelitis and significant soft tissue compromise.

amputation has been documented at 50% to 60% in this population, efforts in nonre-constructive and reconstructive surgical intervention should be exhausted before definitive amputation.[44] Fortunately, advances in staged amputation planning and use of targeted muscle reinnervation have greatly improved lower extremity rehabili-tation and postoperative function outcomes when amputation is required.[45,46]

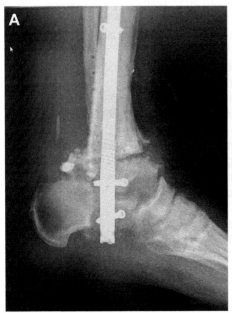
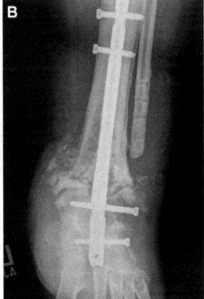

Fig. 6. (*A, B*) A patient with nonreconstructable deformity secondary to prior charcot arthropathy and attempted reconstruction. Due to the extent of bone necrosis and hard-ware failure, patients may benefit from below knee amputation and early rehabilitation with prosthesis as opposed to repeated attempts at salvage.

SUMMARY

Nonreconstructive surgeries have their role to preventing progression or sequelae of Charcot arthropathy for those who have failed nonoperative care. Careful patient selection and considering the aforementioned considerations before proceeding with surgical management of Charcot have demonstrated good outcomes. Nonreconstructive surgeries such as ostectomies, external fixation, soft tissue releases and soft tissue balancing may be sufficient to treating a complex Charcot deformity while avoiding a major midfoot or hindfoot reconstructive surgery as well as proximal limb loss that are not without their own set of risks and complications.

DISCLOSURE

The authors have nothing to disclose regarding conflict of interest or commercial relationship related to the content of this article.

REFERENCES

1. Wukich DK, Sung W, Wipf SA, et al. The consequences of complacency: managing the effects of unrecognized Charcot feet. Diabet Med 2011;28(2):195–8.
2. Smith C, Kumar S, Causby R. The effectiveness of non-surgical interventions in the treatment of Charcot foot. Int J Evid Based Healthc 2007;5(4):437–49.
3. Smith F, Dryburgh N, Donaldson J, et al. Debridement for surgical wounds. Cochrane Database Syst Rev 2013;9. https://doi.org/10.1002/14651858. CD006214.pub4.
4. Janis JE, Kwon RK, Attinger CE. The new reconstructive ladder: modifications to the traditional model. Plast Reconstr Surg 2011;127(Suppl 1):205S–12S.
5. Sohn M-W, Lee TA, Stuck RM, et al. Mortality risk of Charcot arthropathy compared with that of diabetic foot ulcer and diabetes alone. Diabetes Care 2009;32(5):816–21.
6. Pakarinen T-K, Laine H-J, Mäenpää H, et al. Long-term outcome and quality of life in patients with Charcot foot. Foot Ankle Surg 2009;15(4):187–91.
7. Wukich DK, Raspovic KM, Hobizal KB, et al. Surgical management of charcot arthropathy of the ankle and hindfoot in patients with diabetes. Diabetes Metab Res Rev 2016;32(Suppl 1):292–6.
8. Donegan R, Sumpio B, Blume PA. Charcot foot and ankle with osteomyelitis. Diabet Foot Ankle 2013;4. https://doi.org/10.3402/dfa.v4i0.21361.
9. Cates NK, Elmarsafi T, Bunka TJ, et al. Peripheral vascular disease diagnostic related outcomes in diabetic charcot reconstruction. J Foot Ankle Surg 2019; 58(6):1058–63.
10. Chang BB, Shah DM, Darling RC 3rd, et al. Treatment of the diabetic foot from a vascular surgeon's viewpoint. Clin Orthop Relat Res 1993;296:27–30. Available at: https://www.ncbi.nlm.nih.gov/pubmed/8222437.
11. Cates NK, Furmanek J, Dubois KS, et al. Risk factors and outcomes after surgical reconstruction of charcot arthropathy in fracture versus dislocation patterns. J Foot Ankle Surg 2021. https://doi.org/10.1053/j.jfas.2021.07.020. Published online July 26.
12. Wukich DK, Crim BE, Frykberg RG, et al. Neuropathy and poorly controlled diabetes increase the rate of surgical site infection after foot and ankle surgery. J Bone Joint Surg Am 2014;96(10):832–9.

13. Elmarsafi T, Anghel EL, Sinkin J, et al. Risk factors associated with major lower extremity amputation after osseous diabetic charcot reconstruction. J Foot Ankle Surg 2019;58(2):295–300.

14. Gil J, Schiff AP, Pinzur MS. Cost comparison: limb salvage versus amputation in diabetic patients with charcot foot. Foot Ankle Int 2013;34(8):1097–9.

15. Brodsky JW, Rouse AM. Exostectomy for symptomatic bony prominences in diabetic charcot feet. Clin Orthop Relat Res 1993;296:21–6. Available at: https://www.ncbi.nlm.nih.gov/pubmed/8222428.

16. Catanzariti AR, Mendicino R, Haverstock B. Ostectomy for diabetic neuroarthropathy involving the midfoot. J Foot Ankle Surg 2000;39(5):291–300.

17. Leventen EO. Charcot foot—a technique for treatment of chronic plantar ulcer by saucerization and primary closure. Foot Ankle 1986;6(6):295–9.

18. Laurinaviciene R, Kirketerp-Moeller K, Holstein PE. Exostectomy for chronic midfoot plantar ulcer in Charcot deformity. J Wound Care 2008;17(2):53–5.

19. Rosenblum BI, Giurini JM, Miller LB, et al. Neuropathic ulcerations plantar to the lateral column in patients with Charcot foot deformity: a flexible approach to limb salvage. J Foot Ankle Surg 1997;36(5):360–3.

20. Belczyk R, Ramanujam CL, Capobianco CM, et al. Combined midfoot arthrodesis, muscle flap coverage, and circular external fixation for the chronic ulcerated Charcot deformity. Foot Ankle Spec 2010;3(1):40–4.

21. Ramanujam CL, Zgonis T. Versatility of intrinsic muscle flaps for the diabetic Charcot foot. Clin Podiatr Med Surg 2012;29(2):323–6, ix.

22. Sato T, Ichioka S. Ostectomy and medial plantar artery flap reconstruction for charcot foot ulceration involving the midfoot. J Foot Ankle Surg 2016;55(3):628–32.

23. Chen L, Greisberg J. Achilles lengthening procedures. Foot Ankle Clin 2009;14(4):627–37.

24. Hastings MK, Mueller MJ, Sinacore DR, et al. Effects of a tendo-Achilles lengthening procedure on muscle function and gait characteristics in a patient with diabetes mellitus. J Orthop Sports Phys Ther 2000;30(2):85–90.

25. Lamm BM, Paley D, Herzenberg JE. Gastrocnemius soleus recession: a simpler, more limited approach. J Am Podiatr Med Assoc 2005;95(1):18–25. Available at: http://www.ncbi.nlm.nih.gov/pubmed/15659410.

26. Greenhagen RM, Johnson AR, Bevilacqua NJ. Gastrocnemius recession or tendo-achilles lengthening for equinus deformity in the diabetic foot? Clin Podiatr Med Surg 2012;29(3):413–24.

27. Hatt RN, Lamphier TA. Triple hemisection: a simplified procedure for lengthening the Achilles tendon. N Engl J Med 1947;236(5):166–9.

28. Hansen ST. Functional reconstruction of the foot and ankle. Lippincott Williams & Wilkins; 2000. Available at: https://play.google.com/store/books/details?id=ASSCGDRC-KsC.

29. Tiruveedhula M, Graham A, Thapar A, et al. Outcomes of Tendo-Achilles lengthening and weight-bearing total contact cast for management of early midfoot charcot arthropathy. J Clin Orthop Trauma 2021;17:128–38.

30. Holthusen SM, Kolodziej P. Midfoot charcot arthropathy with improvement of arch after achilles tendon lengthening: a case report. Foot Ankle Int 2009;30(9):891–4.

31. Laborde JM. Midfoot ulcers treated with gastrocnemius-soleus recession. Foot Ankle Int 2009;30(9):842–6.

32. Laborde JM, Philbin TM, Chandler PJ, et al. Preliminary results of primary gastrocnemius-soleus recession for midfoot charcot arthropathy. Foot Ankle Spec 2016;9(2):140–4.

33. Ho T. Tendon transfers for chronic ulcerations in diabetics. Available at: http://images3.podiatrym.com/pdf/2019/11/Giurini1119Web.pdf. Accessed June 21, 2022.

34. McKittrick LS, McKittrick JB, Risley TS. Transmetatarsal amputation for infection or gangrene in patients with diabetes mellitus. Ann Surg 1949;130(4):826–42.

35. Boffeli TJ, Tabatt JA. Minimally invasive early operative treatment of progressive foot and ankle deformity associated with charcot-marie-tooth disease. J Foot Ankle Surg 2014. https://doi.org/10.1053/j.jfas.2014.03.019. Published online August 14.

36. Garceau GJ, Palmer RM. Transfer of the anterior tibial tendon for recurrent club foot. J Bone Joint Surg 1967;49(2):207–332.

37. Ober FR. Tendon transplantation in the lower extremity. N Engl J Med 1933; 209(2):52–9.

38. Watkins MB, Jones JB, Ryder CT, et al. Transplantation of the posterior tibial tendon. J Bone Joint Surg 1954;36(6):1181–9.

39. Wagenaar F-CBM, Louwerens JWK. Posterior tibial tendon transfer: results of fixation to the dorsiflexors proximal to the ankle joint. Foot Ankle Int 2007;28(11): 1128–42.

40. Pinzur MS. Neutral ring fixation for high-risk nonplantigrade Charcot midfoot deformity. Foot Ankle Int 2007;28(9):961–6.

41. Cooper PS. Application of external fixators for management of Charcot deformities of the foot and ankle. Foot Ankle Clin 2002;7(1):207–54.

42. Farber DC, Juliano PJ, Cavanagh PR, et al. Single stage correction with external fixation of the ulcerated foot in individuals with charcot arthropathy. Foot Ankle Int 2002;23(2):130–4.

43. Paola LD, Ceccacci T, Ninkovic S, et al. Limb salvage in charcot foot and ankle osteomyelitis: combined use single stage/double stage of arthrodesis and external fixation. Foot Ankle Int 2009;30(11):1065–70.

44. Meshkin DH, Zolper EG, Chang K, et al. Long-term mortality after nontraumatic major lower extremity amputation: a systematic review and meta-analysis. J Foot Ankle Surg 2020. https://doi.org/10.1053/j.jfas.2020.06.027. Published online September 3.

45. Chang BL, Attinger CE, Akbari CM, et al. Targeted muscle reinnervation reduces pain and improves ambulation in patients undergoing below-knee amputation: a single-institution matched cohort study. J Vasc Surg 2020;72(1):e30–1.

46. Carroll PJ, Ragothaman K, Mayer A, et al. Ankle disarticulation: an underutilized approach to staged below knee amputation—case series and surgical technique. J Foot Ankle Surg 2020;59(4):869–72.

Nondiabetic Charcot Neuroarthropathy
Evaluation and Treatment

Emily C. Wagler, DPM

KEYWORDS

- Nondiabetic Charcot neuroarthropathy (CN) • Nondiabetic Charcot reconstruction
- Nondiabetic Charcot treatment

KEY POINTS

- Many underlying causes of nondiabetic Charcot neuroarthropathy (CN) result in poor bone quality.
- Treatment of the nondiabetic CN should be aimed at optimizing bone health and healing, whether medical or surgical.
- The most robust fixation possible should be used in nondiabetic CN reconstruction.

HISTORY OF CHARCOT NEUROARTHROPATHY

Diabetic neuropathy is the most common cause of Charcot neuroarthropathy (CN) in the developed world[1–3]; however, any condition that can cause peripheral neuropathy can cause CN (**Tables 1**).[4,5] Historically, neuropathic joint changes were caused by nondiabetic causes. Venereal diseases, leprosy, and rheumatism were some of the first known associations with neuroarthropathy,[17–20] but it was Jean-Marie Charcot's study of arthropathy and tabes dorsalis that established neuroarthropathy as a distinct pathologic entity in 1881.[17,18,20,20] W.R. Jordan established the correlation between diabetes and arthropathic foot and ankle pathology in 1936,[20] and presently diabetes remains the most common cause in the development of CN.[17]

Causes of Nondiabetic Charcot Neuroarthropathy

There are numerous nondiabetic causes of CN; these can be further categorized into infectious, traumatic, metabolic, inflammatory, medication-induced, congenital/genetic/other, and idiopathic causes of CN. Examples of each category are listed in **Table 1**.[20,21,22]

Department of Podiatry and Foot & Ankle Surgery, The Vancouver Clinic, 501 Southeast 172nd Avenue, Vancouver, WA 98684, USA
E-mail address: ecwagler@gmail.com

Clin Podiatr Med Surg 39 (2022) 571–584
https://doi.org/10.1016/j.cpm.2022.05.004
0891-8422/22/© 2022 Elsevier Inc. All rights reserved.

Table 1
Various nondiabetic causes of Charcot neuroarthropathy

Infectious	Traumatic	Metabolic	Inflammatory	Medications	Congenital/Genetic/Other
Amyloidosis	Cerebrovascular accident (CVA)	Alcoholism	Lupus	Chemotherapeutic agents	Charcot-Marie-Tooth
Human immunodeficiency virus (HIV)	Peripheral nerve injury	Nutritional deficiencies (eg, vitamin B12)	Rheumatoid arthritis	Chronic corticosteroids	Spina bifida
Leprosy	Spinal cord injury	Pernicious anemia	Sjögren syndrome	HIV medications	Syringomyelia
Tabes dorsalis	—	—	—	Toxins	—

Any disease or pathology that can cause neuropathy can potentially cause CN. Tabes dorsalis is a complication of tertiary syphilis and was one of the first identified causes of neuroarthropathy. This neurosyphilis disease primarily affects the posterior roots of the spinal cord and can cause nerve degeneration and progressive joint destruction.[23] Human immunodeficiency virus (HIV)-associated neuropathy can either be a direct cause of HIV infection or neurotoxicity from antiretroviral treatments or a combination of both. Although the exact cause of primary HIV-induced neuropathy is unknown, neuronal injury is likely caused by macrophage dysfunction, overproduction of proinflammatory cytokines, or by the HIV-1 envelope protein gp120.[10] Although not infective, inflammatory arthropathies such as rheumatoid arthritis and Lupus similarly exhibit an overactive inflammatory response, inhibiting osteoblast formation, inducing osteoclast activity, and ultimately leading to bone and joint destruction. In addition, rheumatoid patients have an incidence of 17% to 57% of some form of peripheral neuropathy.[12] Leprosy, or Hansen disease, is caused by Mycobacterium leprae, which is known to have an affinity for peripheral nerves, especially the tibial nerve.[24] Neurotoxicity that can cause peripheral neuropathy is a known complication of alcoholism, many HIV medications, chemotherapeutic agents, toxins, and certain vitamin deficiencies.[7,25–27] It is thought that the reduction in bone mineral density and analgesic effect to damaged joints can cause CN in patients on chronic corticosteroids.[27] Lastly, central or peripheral nervous system pathology can arise from direct trauma or cerebrovascular accident, or congenital or genetic diseases such as spina bifida[15] or Charcot-Marie-Tooth, all of which have been shown to cause peripheral neuropathy.[20] There are many case reports of nondiabetic CN in the literature and are discussed in a later section.

Incidence and Prevalence

The literature is inconsistent in defining the incidence and prevalence of diabetic CN. Many sources agree the incidence may be as low as 0.1%, but one study by Cofield and colleagues[28] found a prevalence of radiographic changes in 29% of diabetic patients with established peripheral neuropathy. In addition, Armstrong reported a prevalence of CN in 0.16% of the general diabetic population but that number increased to 13% of high-risk diabetic patients presenting to a diabetic foot clinic.[29] The exact incidence of CN is further confounded by a high rate of missed or delayed diagnosis,[20] which occurs in close to 25% of patients.[30–32] There are no known studies that report the incidence of nondiabetic CN, but it is likely even more underreported than diabetic CN due to lack of a diagnostic hint from a diabetes diagnosis.

Patient Workup: History of Present Illness

Patient evaluation in nondiabetic CN is similar to diabetic CN with a few important distinctions. Firstly, because diabetic CN is reliant on clinical presentation and a high index of suspicion is incredibly valuable, a very thorough history is necessary with special attention to any history of neuropathy or neuropathy causing diseases and trauma,[33] although one study found only 22% of patients were able to identify a specific trauma.[33,34] When evaluating a nondiabetic patient with suspected CN, the underlying cause is important to identify, as it may alter the course of treatment. A thorough history of past and present medications may reveal chronic steroid use or history of chemotherapy or highly active antiretroviral therapy treatment. A social history may reveal excessive alcohol intake. As with diabetic CN, it is very important to elucidate any history of past or present ulcerations or infections in the foot and ankle and understand that nondiabetic CN may also mimic infection or occur alongside infection.[33] A patient's social history can be just as important as past medical history.

The author recommends that tobacco use, whether smoked or smokeless, alcohol abuse, and any history of drug abuse should be documented with the goal of complete cessation before any surgical reconstruction. In addition, if treatment includes any period of non–weight-bearing, it is important to elucidate the patient's social support (family, friends), ascertain information about their living situation, including type of home or residence and number of stairs, and discuss the patient's ability to navigate their home with a non–weight-bearing limb. The contralateral limb must also be evaluated for the presence of wounds or evidence of Charcot breakdown and should be able to bear weight safely during the period of non–weight-bearing in the affected limb.

Patient Workup: Physical Examination

Even if there is a known cause of the neuropathy, a full neurologic examination (Semmes Weinstein 5.07 monofilament, sharp/dull discrimination, position sense, clonus, patellar, and Achilles reflexes [Wilson]) should be completed, and a referral to a neurologist may be prudent, especially if the neuropathy is thought to be idiopathic. It is also important to perform a proper vascular examination, as more recent literature documents rates of peripheral vascular disease (PAD) as high as 40% in patients with diabetic CN.[35] When optimizing diabetic patients with CN for surgery, Raspovic and colleagues[36] recommend performing a Doppler examination and noninvasive vascular studies on all patients with CN, even if pulses are palpable. If any of the studies are abnormal, a vascular surgery referral is recommended, especially if surgical intervention is planned. One study of diabetic patients with CN after reconstruction found that patients diagnosed with PAD via angiography compared with clinically had a higher rate of return to ambulation and a trend toward lower rate of major amputation.[6] Although this was a study of diabetic patients, the threshold for vascular referral should still be low in nondiabetic patients undergoing CN reconstruction. The physical examination should also include a weight-bearing examination, if deemed safe for the patient, as well as evaluation of limb length, joint range of motion, reducibility of the deformities, and any soft tissue contractures.[36]

Patient Workup: Diagnostics

Diagnosing CN in a nondiabetic patient may prove challenging. Even if a patient denies a history of diabetes, the author always recommends testing hemoglobin A1c (HbA1c). In their article discussing optimization before diabetic CN reconstruction, Raspovic and colleagues outline a preoperative checklist. Similar to diabetic CN, infection must always be ruled out in nondiabetic CN. Infection laboratories should include a complete blood cell count (CBC), erythrocyte sedimentation rate (ESR), and C-reactive protein (CRP).[36] Vitamin D is a critical component of bone healing and can increase the risk of delayed or nonunion in foot and ankle surgery 8 times when insufficient or deficient[37]; this is especially important when evaluating a nondiabetic patient with CN, as many of the nondiabetic CN causes, such as chronic steroid use[38,39] or alcohol abuse,[7,40] are known to have an antagonistic effect on bone health. Whether the patient is diabetic or not, weight-bearing foot and ankle radiographs should be taken and should include a hindfoot alignment view. Advanced imaging can also be helpful; an MRI can be used to identify affected joints that may not show radiographic changes, and a CT may aid in 3-dimensional planning for operative intervention.[36] One study found that in clinically asymptomatic feet in patients with leprosy, 9 out of 10 patients had MRI changes consistent with joint degradation and synovitis. The investigators concluded that MRI may play a role in detecting feet at risk in a neuropathic patient.[41] It is important to note that MRI and even technetium bone scans can lead to false positives for osteomyelitis, especially in the acute phase of Charcot,[42] and must be analyzed with caution.

Clinics Care Points: Patient Workup

- A full neurologic workup is recommended and a neurology referral is prudent in cases of neuropathy with an unknown cause.
- Always rule out infection.
- Properly assess vascular status, especially in preoperative patients.
- HbA1c should always be checked if no recent results are available.
- Vitamin D should also be checked.
- Advanced imaging (CT or MRI) may be helpful for surgical planning but MRI has been shown to lead to false-positive results for osteomyelitis.

Treatment: Medical

Charcot bone is fractured bone, and osseous healing is necessary even if operative treatment is not planned. Nondiabetic patients with CN were found to have a 16 times high delayed union rate in a recent comparative study between nondiabetic and diabetic patients with CN undergoing reconstruction[6]; therefore, bone healing optimization is critical in the nondiabetic patient with CN. There are many ways to optimize bone healing potential in the nondiabetic patient with CN, and it is recommended to consider obtaining the following laboratory findings even if planned treatment is nonoperative. Even if the patient claims they are not diabetic, it is prudent to obtain a new HbA1c (unless recently tested and was less than 6.5). Vitamin 25-hydroxyvitamin D (vitamin D) is a critical component of bone healing. Raspovic and colleagues[36] recommend 50,000 units once weekly for 12 weeks for serum 25-hydroxyvitamin D less than 30 ng/mL in prereconstruction patients. Patients with vitamin D deficiency are 8.1 times more likely to develop nonunion.[37] If there is a history of a wound or infection is suspected, obtain CBC, ESR, and CRP.[36] If reconstruction is planned, the author recommends obtaining parathyroid hormone (PTH) and thyroid stimulating hormone (TSH) levels. Teriparatide, which is synthetic/recombinant human parathyroid hormone, has been shown to improve fusion rates in complex foot and ankle arthrodesis[43] and also in a case report of nonunion after CN reconstruction.[44] Biphosphonates may also improve resolution time in CN patients with acute CN. The investigators of a systematic review recommend the use of bisphosphonates (in the absence of renal insufficiency) at the physician's discretion in acute CN cases that are recalcitrant to immobilization. They found level II evidence that supports bisphosphonate use but also cited level II evidence that bisphosphonates do not improve resolution time.[45,46] Intranasal calcitonin has been shown to reduce bone turnover in patients with CN. In contrast to bisphosphonate therapy, calcitonin is not contraindicated in patients with renal insufficiency.[47] A randomized controlled trial showed 200 IU daily of intranasal calcitonin reduced bone turnover in the first 3 months of treatment of patients with acute CN.[47] Because first-line treatment of acute CN usually requires several months of immobilization, it is critical to consider deep vein thrombosis (DVT) prophylaxis. DVT prophylaxis is recommended in any patient with an immobilized lower limb. A recent prospective found 25% of low-risk patients who underwent elective foot and ankle surgery had a DVT via ultrasonography. Thirty percent of these were found 6 weeks postoperatively and 75% had no clinical symptoms[48] DVT prophylaxis is recommended in patients with lower limb immobilization, and this is confirmed by 2 systematic reviews[49,50] and a meta-analysis.[51] Whether or not operative treatment is planned, many of the aforementioned laboratory tests and medical treatment may help improve outcomes and osseous healing in the nondiabetic patient with CN.

Treatment: Nonsurgical

Patient selection and optimization for nondiabetic CN reconstruction are similar to that of diabetic CN with a few additional areas of consideration. Regardless of cause, the goals of treatment of CN are to maintain or create a stable foot and ankle, avoid ulceration and infection, and preserve a plantigrade foot.[33] Pain that interferes with activities of daily life is also an indication for CN treatment and is often operative.[36] Nondiabetic neuropathy has been found to be vastly underestimated and can have a large negative impact on quality of life.[52] Nonsurgical treatment is very similar to nonsurgical treatment of acute diabetic CN and primarily consists of offloading. Offloading is usually considered the gold standard and has been shown to be safe in neuropathic, diabetic patients with CN.[53,54] The medium time patients spend in a total contact cast is 4 months.[54] Special considerations for the nondiabetic patient with CN must include a patient's ability to safely comply with non–weight-bearing treatment and casting, as many of the causes of nondiabetic CN are shown to reduce bone mineral density and a fall due to instability could result in a hip fracture or other fracture. One study showed that 48% of geriatric fractures occurred due to accident/environment and gait instability/weakness[55]; this is important in the nondiabetic CN population, as one large study had an average age of 75.9 years for nondiabetic patients with CN.[22]

Treatment: Surgical

There is no known literature that focuses on specific operative treatments of nondiabetic CN, but many articles include information on operative reconstruction. As with diabetic CN reconstruction, it is advisable to follow the superconstruct principles in nondiabetic CN reconstruction. Because of the inherently dissolute, fractured, and dislocated bone in patients with CN, a surgeon must rely on fixation devices that do not follow traditional orthopedic principles.[42] Sammarco introduces these 4 principles in 2008, and they are summarized as follows: (1) extension of fixation beyond the zone of injury and affected joints, (2) reducing skin tension as well as the deformity by shortening and removing bone, (3) utilization of the strongest hardware and devices possible, as allowed by the patient's soft tissue and anatomy, and (4) application of fixation devices in the strongest possible position and location.[42] These principles become especially important in the nondiabetic patient with CN, which, as previously discussed, may be even more predisposed to abnormal bone mineral density due to the underlying CN cause[27] and have been found to have increased rates of delayed union.[6] Biomechanical analyses have found screw fixation quality reduces with decreasing bone mineral density.[56,57] Osteoporosis, poor bone mineral density, and soft tissue compromise have long been indications for the use of external fixation[58–60] and may be extremely advantageous in the nondiabetic patient with CN. Similarly, intramedullary nails can be indicated for use in osteoporotic bone, and specifically, a retrograde intramedullary nail from the calcaneus into the talus and tibia may reduce soft tissue dissection and in some cases allow for earlier weight-bearing.[61,62] Both fixation constructs have been widely used in CN reconstruction, and the simultaneous use of both intramedullary nail and circular external fixation for bone defects[63] and specifically CN reconstruction has been described in the literature.[64] In addition, locking plates and intramedullary beams are indicated in osteoporotic bone and do follow superconstruct principles.[42] Although studied only in the diabetic CN population, internal fixation combined with external fixation in CN reconstruction can provide a very robust construct and high rates of limb salvage.[65] Although the literature describing CN fixation constructs focuses on primarily diabetic patients, it is important to consider a combined internal (whether it is locking plates, beams, or intramedullary nails) and external fixation construct in nondiabetic CN reconstruction, given their propensity to have low bone mineral density and increased delayed union rates.[6] Although, even with a high likelihood of poor bone stock, nondiabetic patients with CN have been shown to be much more likely to return to ambulation after reconstruction compared with their diabetic CN counterparts.[6]

Clinics Care Points: Treatment

- Bone healing optimization is crucial in both surgical and nonsurgical nondiabetic patients with CN.
- Nondiabetic patients with CN are at higher risk for developing delayed union and may be prone to poor bone quality due to their underlying neuropathic cause.
- Bisphosphonates may improve resolution time in active CN but are contraindicated in patients with renal disease. Calcitonin is safe in renal impairment and has been shown to reduce bone turnover.
- DVT prophylaxis is recommended in any nondiabetic patient with CN with non–weight-bearing as part of their treatment.
- Fall prevention in nondiabetic patients with CN is essential, and many of these patients may have reduced bone density and are predisposed to fragility fractures.
- Superconstruct principles should be used in nondiabetic CN reconstruction, and the employment of intramedullary nails or external fixation is advised due to their propensity of poor bone stock and delayed union.
- Bone stimulation has been shown to be beneficial after reconstruction and is recommended in the nondiabetic patient with CN.

Research

The literature for nondiabetic CN is relatively sparse compared with diabetic CN, and there are no known level I or II studies that focused on nondiabetic CN. Most nondiabetic CN literature exists as small case reports or case series with a few larger comparative studies.[6] Case series of nondiabetic CN of the foot and ankle are summarized in **Table 2**. Syringomyelia was intentionally excluded from the table, as there are no known cases causing CN of the foot or ankle in a recent literature review.[66]

The largest known study reporting nondiabetic CN was by Bariteau and colleagues.[22] This retrospective case series investigated 59 patients over a period of 23 years, and the average follow-up was 60 months. The average age of patients was 75.9 years, and all patients were found to have idiopathic neuropathy, and the study excluded any patients with a known cause of peripheral neuropathy, including, but not limited to, diabetes, rheumatoid arthritis, toxin exposure, and chemotherapy. A CN diagnosis was made clinically and neuropathy established by the inability to feel a Semmes-Weinstein 5.07 mm monofilament. The patients were not noted to have undergone exhaustive evaluation by a neurologist. The researchers categorized radiographs using the Brodsky anatomic classification. Treatment was based on the Eichenholtz classification, with stage I patients undergoing total contact casting, and those with persistent ulceration and/or nonplantigrade or nonbraceable feet went on to surgical reconstruction. Forty-six patients underwent operative intervention, and at last follow-up, 38 of these patients were ambulatory. Of the remaining patients, 6 had persistent ulceration and 2 patients with ankle CN required below-knee amputation. The investigators noted that the operative rate was higher (50%)

Table 2
Case series of nondiabetic Charcot neuroarthropathy of the foot and ankle

Cause	Author	Number of Patients
Alcoholic neuropathy	Cates 2020[6]	4
Alcoholic neuropathy	Shibuya[7]	4
Amiodarone	Dhatariya[8]	1
Charcot-Marie-Tooth	Cates 2020[6]	2
Herpetic encephalitis	Shinjo[9]	1
HIV neuropathy	Young[10]	1
Leprosy	Rostom[11]	2
Lupus	Cates 2020[6]	1
Poststroke	Cates 2020[6]	1
Rheumatoid arthritis	Grear[12]	14
Sjögren syndrome	Nguyen[13]	1
Spina bifida	Yalcin[14]	5
Spina bifida	Nagarkatti[15]	10
Steroid use	Cates 2020[6]	2
Vincristine	McKay[16]	1

compared with a comparable group of operative diabetic patients with CN (40%), and the transtibial amputation rate for foot CN was zero in the nondiabetic group.[22,67]

The most recent study and largest cohort of nondiabetic CN undergoing osseous reconstruction was by Cates and colleagues[6,68] in 2020; this was a level III retrospective study that compared matched cohorts of 50 diabetic and 25 nondiabetic patients with CN that underwent osseous reconstruction over a 16-year period. The average age at time of repair was 56 in both groups. Although the diabetic controls were found to have a significantly higher chance of having a preoperative ulcer ($P = .0499$), there were no other significant differences in comorbidities between the 2 groups. Multivariate logistic regression of the postreconstruction outcomes showed that the nondiabetic cohort was 17.6 times more likely to return to ambulation but 16.4 times more likely to develop delayed osseous union, compared with the diabetic cohort. A subanalysis was then performed, matching well-controlled (HbA1c less than or equal to 6.5) diabetics with CN and the nondiabetic patients with CN. Bivariate analysis revealed the well-controlled diabetic CN group had higher rates of renal disease, including end-stage renal disease and preoperative ulceration, and the nondiabetic CN group was significantly more likely to return to ambulation ($P = .0153$) and develop a delayed osseous union ($P = .0202$). However, when multivariate analysis was performed, only return to ambulation was significant. The investigators theorize the lower rate of return to ambulation in the diabetic CN cohort was multifactorial but closely related to preoperative ulceration. They suggest the lower rate of ambulation may be related to prolonged non–weight-bearing period in the presence of an ulcer, difficulty ambulating due to previous surgical treatment of foot and ankle infections, and overall decreased walking capacity in the presence of a plantar ulceration. The investigators also discuss the increased rate of delayed osseous union in the nondiabetic CN cohort, which is closely related to the underlying cause of the nondiabetic CN. Many of the causes of neuropathy in this study were found to correlate with decreased bone mineral density. Interestingly, when comparing the nondiabetic CN cohort with well-controlled diabetics, the rate of delayed osseous union was not significantly different. The investigators theorize this may be due to osteoprotective benefits of both insulin and metformin.[6]

Overall, the literature for nondiabetic CN is sparse with very few larger studies and no level I or level II evidence. Although there are many case reports and case series, there is a deficit of larger comparative studies of nondiabetic patients with CN.

Complications and Concerns Unique to Nondiabetic Charcot Neuroarthropathy

Treatment of diabetic and nondiabetic CN can be a challenging and complicated process for both the patient and provider. Diabetic patients with CN can develop comorbidities associated with prolonged hyperglycemia such as renal disease, vascular disease, and immune compromise. However, nondiabetic patients with CN can have their own unique complications and treatment concerns. In their study comparing diabetic and nondiabetic patients with CN after reconstruction, Cates and colleagues[6] illustrated that nondiabetic patients with CN were at much greater risk of delayed osseous union. This study elucidates that many of the underlying causes of nondiabetic peripheral neuropathy can also be associated with reduced bone mineral density and poor bone quality, which puts nondiabetic patients with CN at greater risk of osseous healing complications. The other large study on nondiabetic CN, by Bariteau and colleagues, reported on a much larger cohort of nondiabetic patients with CN, with those patients having an average age of 75.9 years. The investigators speculate this is due to the longer period of time involved in developing idiopathic neuropathy. However, this can also introduce an increased incidence and prevalence of PAD, as this has been shown to sharply increase in a patient's 60s and 70s.[69] Although the presence of PAD has been proved to no longer be inhibitive of CN development, it can certainly negatively affect wound healing and reconstruction outcomes.[35,68] Further research is necessary to establish a correlation between nondiabetic CN and increased rates of PAD compared with diabetic CN.

Treatment Recommendations

1. Obtain a neurology consult if there is no known cause of the neuropathy
2. Use total contact cast in the acute phase[53,54]
3. Recommend HbA1c (unless recently tested and was less than 6.5) and vitamin D
4. If there is a history of a wound or infection is suspected, obtain CBC, ESR, and CRP[36]
5. Optimize bone healing potential: laboratory findings
   a. Recommend 50,000 units of vitamin D once weekly for 12 weeks for serum 25-hydroxyvitamin D less than 30 ng/mL in prereconstruction patients[36]
   b. If reconstruction if planned, also obtain PTH and TSH levels
6. Optimize bone heal potential: medical treatment
   a. Teriparatide has been shown to improve fusion rates in complex foot and ankle arthrodesis[43,44]
   b. Biphosphonates may improve resolution time in acute patients with acute CN but are contraindicated in renal insufficiency and some studies say are ineffective in improving acute CN resolution time[45,46]
   c. Intranasal calcitonin has been shown to reduce bone turnover and is not contraindicated in patients with renal insufficiency[47]
7. DVT prophylaxis is recommended in any patient with and immobilized lower limb[48–51]

8. The surgical indications for nondiabetic patients with CN are the same as diabetic patients with CN: chronic CN and persistent joint instability and/or severe deformity despite proper conservative management[46]
9. Surgical treatment and reconstruction should follow superconstruct principles[42]
   a. External fixation and intramedullary beams or nails should be used when possible, especially in the presence of poor bone stock of the nondiabetic patient with CN
10. Consider use of electrical bone stimulation in all postreconstruction patients
    a. Nondiabetic CN reconstruction patients are at even higher risk of delayed union[6]
    b. Has been shown to be safe and effective in CN reconstruction[70]
11. Depending on cause and patient workup, nondiabetic patients with CN may be better surgical candidates than a comorbid diabetic patient with CN, so they are more likely to benefit from reconstruction (more likely to ambulate and more likely to undergo surgical correction)

SUMMARY

Nondiabetic CN is an uncommon pathology and likely missed or delayed in diagnosis. However, a physician who treats CN is likely to encounter the nondiabetic patient with CN. Although there are many similarities between nondiabetic and diabetic CN, many of the underlying causes causing nondiabetic neuropathy and CN are associated with poor bone quality. Further, nondiabetic patients with CN have been shown to have delayed bone healing after reconstruction compared with diabetic patients with CN. Therefore, robust fixation is encouraged when reconstructing the nondiabetic patient with CN. Treatment options and workup for the nondiabetic patients with CN are similar to those for diabetic patients with CN but special consideration and even treatment should be given to optimize bone healing, even in a nonoperative patient. Lastly, nondiabetic patients with CN have been shown to have much higher rates of return to ambulation after reconstruction compared with diabetic patients with CN and may benefit more from reconstruction than a comorbid diabetic patient with CN.

ACKNOWLEDGMENTS

The author would like to thank Dr Byron Hutchinson for inspiration and passion to treat Charcot as well as the opportunity to contribute to this Clinics issue.

DISCLOSURE

The author does not have any commercial or financial conflicts of interest or funding of any kind.

DISCLOSURE

The author has nothing to disclose.

REFERENCES

1. Johnson-Lynn S, McCaskie A, Coll A, et al. Neuroarthropathy in diabetes: pathogenesis of Charcot arthropathy. Bone Joint Res 2018;7:373–8.
2. Rogers L, Frykberg R, Armstrong D, et al. The Charcot foot in diabetes. Diabetes Care 2011;34:2123–9.

3. Kaynak G, Birsel O, Guven M, et al. An overview of the Charcot foot pathophysiology. Diabetic Foot Ankle 2013;4:1–9.
4. Schneekloth B, Lowery N, Wukich D. Charcot neuroarthropathy in patients with diabetes: an updated systematic review of surgical management. J Foot Ankle Surg 2016;55:586–90.
5. Strotman P, Reif T, Pinzur M. Charcot arthropathy of the foot and ankle. Foot Ankle Int 2016;37:1255–63.
6. Cates N, Wagler E, Bunka T, et al. Charcot reconstruction: outcomes in patients with and without diabetes. J Foot Ankle Surg 2020;59(6):1229–33.
7. Shibuya N, La Fontaine J, Frania S. Alcohol-induced neuroarthropathy in the foot: a case series and review of literature. J Foot Ankle Surg 2008;47:118–24.
8. Dhatariya K, Gooday C, Murchison R, et al. Pedal neuroarthropathy in a nondiabetic patient as a result of long-term amiodarone use. J Foot Ankle Surg 2009; 48(3):362–4.
9. Shinjo S, de Carvalho J. Charcot's arthropathy secondary to herpetic encephalitis sequelae: an unusual presentation. Rheumatol Int 2010;30:973–5.
10. Young N, et al. HIV neuropathy induced charcot neuroarthropathy: a case discussion. Foot 2012;22(3):112–6.
11. Rostom S, Bahiri R, Mahfoud-filali S, et al. Neurogenic osteoarthropathy in leprosy. Clin Rheumatol 2007;26:2153–5.
12. Grear B, Rabinovich A, Brodsky J. Charcot arthropathy of the foot and ankle associated with rheumatoid arthritis. Foot Ankle Int 2013;34(11):1541–7.
13. Nguyen M, Peschken CA. Severe sensory neuronopathy in primary Sjogren syndrome resulting in Charcot arthropathy. J Rheumatol 2016;43(7):1449–51.
14. Yalcin S, Kocaoglu B, Berker N, et al. Conservative treatment of Charcot arthropathy in a series of spina bifida patients: the experience of one center and review of the literature. J Pediatr Orthop B 2007;16(5):373–9.
15. Nagarkatti D, Banta J, Thomson J. Charcot arthropathy in spina bifida. J Pediatr Orthop 2000;20(1):82–7.
16. McKay D, Sheehan P, DeLauro T, et al. Vincristine-induced neuroarthropathy (Charcot's joint). J Am Podiatr Med Assoc 2000;90(9):478–80.
17. Armstrong D, Peters E. Charcot's arthropathy of the foot. Int Diabetes Monitor 2001;13(5):1–5.
18. Jeffcoate W, Lima J, Nobrega L. The Charcot foot. Diabet Med 1999;17:253–8.
19. Fryberg R, Belczyk R. Epidemiology of the charcot foot. Clin Podiatr Med Surg 2008;25:17–28.
20. Sanders L. The Charcot foot: historical perspective 1827–2003. Diabetes Metab Res Rev 2004;20(1):S4–8.
21. Standaert C, Cardenas D, Anderson P. Charcot spine as a late complication of traumatic spinal cord injury. Arch Phys Med Rehabil 1997;78:221–5.
22. Bariteau J, Tenenbaum S, Rabinovich A, et al. Charcot arthropathy of the foot and ankle in patients with idiopathic neuropathy. Foot Ankle Int 2014;35:996–1001.
23. Tatu L, Bogousslavsky J. Tabes dorsalis in the 19th century. The golden age of progressive locomotor ataxia. Rev Neurol (Paris) 2021;177(4):376–84.
24. Moonot P, Ashwood N, Lockwood D. Orthopaedic complications of leprosy. J Bone Joint Surg Br 2005;87:1328–32.
25. Arapostathi C, Tentolouris N, Jude E. Charcot foot associated with chronic alcohol abuse. Case Rep 2013;2013.
26. Kruger M, Nell T. Bone mineral density in people living with HIV: a narrative review of the literature. AIDS Res Ther 2017;14:35.

27. Gilliland B. Neuropathic joint disease in relapsing polychondritis and other arthritides. In: Fauci A, Braunwald E, Isselbacher K, et al, editors. Harrison's principles of internal medicine, 2, 14th edition. New York: McGraw-Hill; 1953. p. 1998.

28. Cofield R, Motrisin M, Beabout J. Diabetic neuroarthropathy in the foot: patient characteristics and patterns of radiographic changes. Foot Ankle Int 1983; 4:5–22.

29. Armstrong D, Todd W, Lavery L, et al. The natural history of acute Charcot's arthropathy in a diabetic foot specialty clinic. Diabet Med 1997;14:357–63.

30. Marks R. Complications of foot and ankle surgery in patients with diabetes. Clin Orthop 2001;391:153–61.

31. Myerson M, Henderson M, Saxby T, et al. Management of midfoot diabetic neuroarthropathy. Foot Ankle Int 1994;15:233–41.

32. Wukich D, Sung W. Charcot arthropathy of the foot and ankle: modern concepts and management review. J Diabet Complications 2009;23(6):409–26.

33. Chantelau E, Richter A, Schmidt-Grigoriadis P, et al. The diabetic Charcot foot: MRI discloses bone stress injury as trigger mechanism of neuroarthropathy. Exp Clin Endocrinol Diabetes 2006;114:118–23.

34. Wilton JP. Lower extremity focused neurologic examination. Clin Podiatr Med Surg 2016;33(2):191–202.

35. Wukich D, Raspovic K, Suder N. Prevalence of peripheral arterial disease in patients with diabetic Charcot neuroarthropathy. J Foot Ankle Surg 2016;55:727–31.

36. Raspovic K, Liu G, Lalli T, et al. Optimizing results in diabetic charcot reconstruction. Clin Podiatr Med Surg 2019;36(3):469–81.

37. Moore K, Howell M, Saltrick K, et al. Risk factors associated with nonunion after elective foot and ankle reconstruction: a case-control study. J Foot Ankle Surg 2017;56(3):457–62.

38. Weinstein R. Glucocorticoid-induced bone disease. N Engl J Med 2011;365: 62–70.

39. Rangel E, Sá J, Gomes S, et al. Charcot neuroarthropathy after simultaneous pancreas-kidney transplant. Transplantation 2012;94:642–5.

40. Turner R. Skeletal response to alcohol. Alcoholism 2000;24:693–1701.

41. Maas M, Slim E, Akkerman E, et al. MRI in clinically asymptomatic neuropathic leprosy feet: a baseline study. Int J Lepr Other Mycobact Dis 2001;69(3):219–24.

42. Sammarco V. Superconstructs in the treatment of charcot foot deformity: plantar plating, locked plating, and axial screw fixation. Foot Ankle Clin 2009;14(3): 393–407.

43. Lee H, Park J, Suh D, et al. Effects of teriparatide on fusion rates in patients undergoing complex foot and ankle arthrodesis. Foot Ankle Surg 2020;26(7): 766–70.

44. Tamai K, Takamatsu K, Kazuki K. Successful treatment of nonunion with teriparatide after failed ankle arthrodesis for Charcot arthropathy. Osteoporos Int 2013; 24:2729–32.

45. Richard J, Almasri M, Schuldiner S. Treatment of acute Charcot foot with bisphosphonates: a systematic review of the literature. Diabetologia 2012;55: 1258–64.

46. Milne T, Rogers J, Kinnear E, et al. Developing an evidence-based clinical pathway for the assessment, diagnosis and management of acute Charcot Neuro-Arthropathy: a systematic review. J Foot Ankle Res 2013;6(1):30.

47. Bem R, Jirkovská A, Fejfarová V, et al. Intranasal calcitonin in the treatment of acute charcot neuroosteoarthropathy. Diabetes Care 2006;29(6):1392–4.

48. Sullivan M, Eusebio ID, Haigh K, et al. Prevalence of deep vein thrombosis in low-risk patients after elective foot and ankle surgery. Foot Ankle Int 2019;40(3):330–5.

49. Testroote M, Stigter W, Janssen L, et al. Low molecular weight heparin for prevention of venous thromboembolism in patients with lower-leg immobilization. In: Testroote M, editor. Cochrane database syst rev, 4. Chichester, UK: John Wiley & Sons Ltd.; 2014. p. CD006681.

50. Zee A, van Lieshout K, van der Heide M, et al. Low molecular weight heparin for prevention of venous thromboembolism in patients with lower-limb immobilization. Cochrane Database Syst Rev 2017;8(8):CD006681.

51. Ettema H, Kollen B, Verheyen C, et al. Prevention of venous thromboembolism in patients with immobilization of the lower extremities: a meta-analysis of randomized controlled trials. J Thromb Haemost 2008;6:1093–8.

52. Brodszky V, Péntek M, Komoly S, et al. Quality of life of patients with non-diabetic peripheral neuropathic pain; results from a cross-sectional survey in general practices in Hungary. Ideggyogy Sz 2015;68(9–10):325–30.

53. de Souza L. Charcot arthropathy and immobilization in a weight-bearing total contact cast. J Bone Joint Surg Am 2008;90(4):754–9.

54. Griffiths D, Kaminski M. Duration of total contact casting for resolution of acute Charcot foot: a retrospective cohort study. J Foot Ankle Res 2021;14(1):44.

55. Rubenstein L. Falls in older people: epidemiology, risk factors and strategies for prevention. Age Ageing 2006;35(2):ii37–41.

56. Stromsoe K, Kok W, Hoiseth A, et al. Holding power of the 4.5 mm AO/ASIF cortex screw in cortical bone in relation to bone mineral density. Injury 1993;24(10):656–9.

57. Trader J, Johnson R, Kalbfleisch J. Bone-mineral content, surface hardness, and mechanical fixation in the human radius. A correlative study. J Bone Joint Surg Am 1979;61(8):217–1220.

58. Beris A, Lykissas M, Sioros V, et al. Femoral periprosthetic fracture in osteoporotic bone after a total knee replacement:treatment with Ilizarov external fixation. J Arthroplasty 2010;25(7):1168.e9.

59. Iliopoulos E, Morrissey N, Cho S, et al. Outcomes of the Ilizarov frame use in elderly patients. J Orthop Sci 2017;22(4):783–6.

60. Ramlee M, Gan H, Daud S, et al. Stress distributions and micromovement of fragment bone of pilon fracture treated with external fixator: a finite element analysis. J Foot Ankle Surg 2020;59(4):664–72.

61. Jordan R, Chapman A, Buchanan D, et al. The role of intramedullary fixation in ankle fractures - a systematic review. Foot Ankle Surg 2018;24(1):1–10.

62. McKean J, Cuellar D, Hak D, et al. Osteoporotic ankle fractures: an approach to operative management. Orthopedics 2013;36(12):936–40.

63. Eralp L, Kocaoglu M, Yusof N, et al. Distal tibial reconstruction with use of a circular external fixator and an intramedullary nail. The combined technique. J Bone Joint Surg Am 2007;89(10):2218–24.

64. Tomczak C, Beaman D, Perkins S. Combined intramedullary nail coated with antibiotic-containing cement and ring fixation for limb salvage in the severely deformed, infected, neuroarthropathic ankle. Foot Ankle Int 2019;40(1):48–55.

65. Hegewald K, Wilder M, Chappell T, et al. Combined internal and external fixation for diabetic charcot reconstruction: a retrospective case series. J Foot Ankle Surg 2016;55(3):619–27.

66. Wang X, Li Y, Gao J, et al. Charcot arthropathy of the shoulder joint as a presenting feature of basilar impression with syringomyelia: a case report and literature review. Medicine (Baltimore) 2018;97(28):e11391.
67. Pinzur M. Surgical versus accommodative treatment for Charcot arthropathy of the midfoot. Foot Ankle Int 2004;25(8):545–9.
68. Cates N, Elmarsafi T, Bunka T, et al. Peripheral vascular disease diagnostic related outcomes in diabetic charcot reconstruction. J Foot Ankle Surg 2019; 58(6):1058–63.
69. Criqui M, Aboyans V. Epidemiology of peripheral artery disease. Circ Res 2015; 116(9):1509–26.
70. Petrisor B, Lau J. Electrical bone stimulation: an overview and its use in high risk and Charcot foot and ankle reconstructions. Foot Ankle Clin 2005;10(4):609–20, vii-viii.

Conservative Management of Charcot Neuroarthropathy

Mallory Schweitzer, DPM, MHA[a],*, Stephen Rockhill, DPM[b]

KEYWORDS

- Charcot neuroarthropathy • Conservative management • Bisphosphonates
- Calcitonin • Immobilization • Nonweight-bearing

KEY POINTS

- Early recognition and initiation of appropriate treatment is important in managing Charcot neuroarthropathy, and the diagnosis can be difficult.
- Conservative treatment includes immobilization and nonweight-bearing until consolidation and stability of the involved joints is achieved.
- Pharmacologic treatments including bisphosphonates, calcitonin, and monoclonal antibodies have been investigated regarding their use in Charcot; however, more research is needed to determine the appropriateness of these medications.

INTRODUCTION

Charcot neuroarthropathy (CN) is a potentially devastating disease that can lead to eventual deformity and morbidity in patients with neuropathy.[1,2] It is characterized by bone and joint destruction that occurs due to trauma, sensory neuropathy, and altered bone metabolism. Sohn and colleagues[1] showed that 34% of patients with CN subsequently develop an ulceration, and this puts patients at higher risk for infection and amputation. Frykberg and colleagues[3] found that the most commonly involved joint is the tarsometatarsal joint (40%); followed by the naviculocuneiform, talonavicular, and calcaneocuboid joints (30%); metatarsophalangeal and interphalangeal joints (15%); and ankle and subtalar joints (10%). Many patients who develop CN are poor surgical candidates, and the quick recognition and appropriate initial treatment can help patients avoid surgical interventions with significant rates of complications.

[a] Multicare Podiatry Associates, 315 M.L.K Jr. Way, Tacoma, WA 98405, USA; [b] Franciscan Foot and Ankle Institute, 34509 9th Avenue South, Federal Way, WA 98003, USA
* Corresponding author.
E-mail address: SchweitzerDPM@gmail.com

Clin Podiatr Med Surg 39 (2022) 585–594
https://doi.org/10.1016/j.cpm.2022.05.005
0891-8422/22/© 2022 Elsevier Inc. All rights reserved.

CLASSIFICATION

The radiographic stages of Charcot are most commonly classified based on a system described by Eichenholtz in 1966.[4] Eichenholtz described Stages 1 to 3, which correlate with radiographic progression from acute fragmentation and deformity of joints to consolidation and resolution of clinical symptoms.[4] Stage 1 is characterized by periarticular debris and fragmentation and joint deformity including subluxation and dislocation. Clinically, the foot seems erythematous and edematous, and there is laxity of the affected ligaments. In Stage 2, the bone begins to consolidate and the foot improves in appearance clinically. Stage 3 represents the reconstitution phase in which fragmented bones and joints consolidate more fully and fibrous ankylosis may also occur. The erythema and edema resolve, and the affected joints may be more stable.[4] In 1990, Shibata described Stage 0 added to this classification, which describes the clinical symptoms that precede the initial positive radiographic findings including erythema, edema, and warmth.[5]

The Brodsky classification is also commonly used, and it describes the anatomic location of the joints affected by CN.[6] The most common type, involving 60% of cases of Charcot, is the midfoot. This includes the naviculocuneiform and tarsometatarsal joints and is classified as type I. Type II includes the subtalar, talonavicular, and calcaneocuboid joints and occurs in 30% to 35% of cases. Involvement of the ankle joint is classified as type IIIA and pathologic fracture of the tuberosity of the calcaneus is type IIIB.[6]

Current classification systems do not include prognostic data or direct clinicians regarding specific treatment options, and new staging systems should be considered to help guide clinical decision-making.[7]

GOALS OF TREATMENT

The recognition of the Charcot process in the prodromal Stage 0 is critical to attempt to prevent the complications associated with progression to deformity. Better functional outcomes have been correlated with correct diagnosis within 3 months of onset.[8] Because the initial symptoms of CN are nonspecific and are easily confused with other clinical entities, it is not uncommon for Charcot to be initially misdiagnosed (**Fig. 1**). The first clinical symptoms include erythema, edema, and warmth, and these are consistent with numerous causes such as infection, trauma, deep vein thrombosis, and inflammatory arthritis.[9] Delayed diagnosis may be devastating for patients who subsequently develop severe nonbraceable deformities with recurrent ulcerations[10,11] (**Fig. 2**). The goals of conservative treatment of Charcot are to maintain a braceable, plantigrade foot without the development of recurrent ulcerations.[7]

CONSERVATIVE TREATMENT

The mainstays of treatment in the acute phase of Charcot are immobilization and nonweight-bearing. Offloading has been described as the most important management strategy in the conservative treatment of Charcot[7] and total contact casts (TCCs) have been described as the gold standard of immobilization. Other devices, such as a removable walker brace and vacuum boot have also been described as appropriate devices for immobilization. Advantages of a TCC include the ability to customize the cast and inability of patients to remove it.[11] If a TCC is used, the cast should be changed frequently to avoid complications such as irritation and ulceration.[7]

However, the length of time of immobilization until resolution of the Charcot process and consolidation varies, and it is difficult to give patients a specific estimate of how

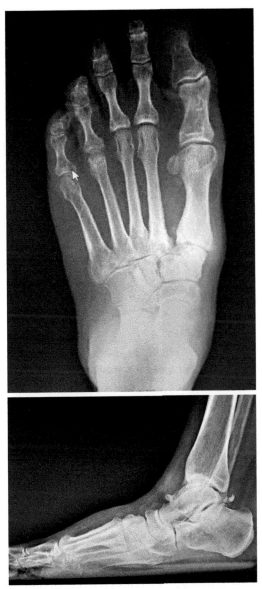

Fig. 1. AP and lateral radiographs of patient who presented for evaluation of cellulitis without open lesions.

long immobilization will be necessary. A review of global population-based studies found the duration of TCC treatment ranging from 3 to 12 months.[9] It has been recommended that casting is continued until there are radiographic signs of consolidation and the temperature differential between the affected and contralateral limb is less than 2°C.

Cases of noncompliance with nonweight-bearing precautions have also been described without progression to significant deformity with only immobilization. Cook and colleagues[12] presented a series of 3 patients who continued weight-

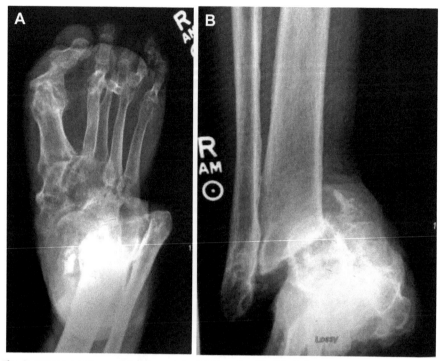

Fig. 2. Severe nonbraceable Charcot foot (*A*) and ankle (*B*) deformity.

bearing despite nonweight-bearing instructions in a vacuum stabilization boot. These patients required immobilization for an average of 90.3 days until the acute Charcot phase resolved and the feet were stable. None of these patients developed significant foot deformities. Every physician treating patients with Charcot has likely encountered certain patients who are noncompliant with nonweight-bearing instructions that do not go on to develop unstable deformity with recurrent ulcerations. As of now, there are no reliable criteria that predict which patients will go on to develop significant deformity if allowed to remain weight-bearing.

CLINICAL MONITORING

Nube and colleagues[13] described the purpose of monitoring CN in patients as 2-fold to include assessing the disease activity as the condition progresses from the acute to chronic phase and identifying structural abnormalities and complications that may arise. This aids the clinician in deciding the duration of primary treatment and helps determine long-term prognosis.[13]

The podiatric clinician should have a high degree of suspicion for CN when evaluating neuropathic patients who present with erythema, edema, and warmth of the foot or ankle. The initial symptoms may be subtle or well localized, in which case regular evaluation is important to avoid mismanagement. Warmth is a well-documented symptom of CN, and the use of handheld infrared temperature scanners has also been advocated, although this is not a common practice for many clinicians.

Radiographic evaluation is also imperative to evaluate patients with this initial presentation. Initial radiographs may be negative or have subtle changes.[14] If there is clinical suspicion for CN with negative initial radiographs, the radiographs should be repeated within several weeks as findings may become more apparent over time.[13]

Because Charcot involves fractures of the affected bones, bone scans or MRI can also be used to detect early disease. However, neither modality is entirely sensitive or specific.[15] Indium 111-labeled white blood cell scans have been recommended in settings where it is necessary to differentiate osteomyelitis from Charcot, although bone biopsy continues to be the gold standard.

PHARMACOLOGIC TREATMENT

There has been increasing interest in pharmacologic treatments that can be used to mitigate the effects of Charcot and shorten the amount of time until osseous consolidation is achieved. Bisphosphonates, calcitonin, and monoclonal antibodies have been investigated to determine the appropriateness and usefulness in cases of Charcot.

BISPHOSPHONATES

Bisphosphonates have been used to treat a variety of skeletal disorders with an excessive osteoclast-mediated bony resorption pathogenesis including osteoporosis, Paget disease, malignancies metastatic to bone, multiple myeloma, and hypercalcemia of malignancy.[16] The utility of bisphosphonates in other osteoclast-mediated disorders has piqued interest in pharmacologic therapy with bisphosphonates in the treatment of CN in the acute phase. There are osteolytic changes that occur in the Charcot foot from unregulated bony resorption, which contributes to the eventual collapse and deformity of the affected bones. Although the exact pathophysiology of CN is not completely understood, current research has focused on the involvement of the receptor activator of nuclear factor-kappa C ligand (RANKL) and osteoprotegerin (OPG) pathway. Recent advancements have shown encouraging information regarding cytokines and their relationship to the RANKL/OPG pathway playing a pivotal role in regards to bone resorption and osteolysis that presents in CN.[17] This occurs by increased interaction between RANKL, nuclear factor kappa-B, and proinflammatory cytokines, such as tumor necrosis factor-alpha, interleukin-1, and interleukin-6, which leads to localized osteolysis that destroys the bone structure.[18] Studies have also shown an increase in bone turnover markers such as carboxyterminal telopeptide of type 1 collagen (1CTP).[19] Therefore, antiresorptive agents such as bisphosphonates, calcitonin, and denosumab have been considered as possible treatment options in combination with immobilization and offloading of the affected Charcot foot.

Pamidronate, a bisphosphonate, has been extensively studied in regards to its use in osteoclast-mediated diseases. It has been shown to decrease the temperature of the Charcot foot and reduce alkaline phosphatase (ALP) concentrations.[20] Pamidronate was also shown to have a positive effect on clinical and radiological improvement.[21] A randomized controlled trial by Jude and colleagues showed a significant decrease in temperature in the Charcot foot in the pamidronate group.[22] With an increase in time, the temperature was not significantly different between the pamidronate and placebo group. Similarly, the pamidronate group showed significant reduction in ALP and urinary dehydroxypyridinoline bone metabolic markers at 4 weeks. At 12 months, the metabolic bone markers normalized to baseline, and there was no statistical difference between the groups. These studies hypothesize that there may be initial short-term benefits that are seen from pamidronate administration.

An oral bisphosphonate, Alendronate, was studied by Pitocco and colleagues.[23] Their study demonstrated significant reduction in bone metabolic markers such as 1CTP and urinary hydroxyproline but not ALP. There was a significant improvement in the bone mineral density of the Charcot foot in the alendronate group compared with the control group. They also reported the visual analog scale was improved in the alendronate group. Pakarinen and colleagues[24] performed a double-blinded randomized placebo-controlled trial with zoledronate. They allowed patients to weight bear when the temperature difference between the 2 feet was less than 1°C for at least 30 days with no evidence of edema or erythema. Their results showed an actual increased median immobilization time in the zoledronate group compared with the placebo group (27 vs 20 weeks). This study demonstrates that the zoledronate group did not have an effect of decreased immobilization time but rather their immobilization time was increased.

Although bisphosphonates may illustrate short-term benefits regarding decrease in temperature, pain, improved radiographic results and decrease in bone metabolic markers in the Charcot foot. There is no significant evidence to suggest that these benefits provide long-term benefits to the Charcot foot and the quality of evidence is relatively low. Many of the studies surrounding bisphosphonates fail to illustrate how limb salvage was affected in the long term, which is an important consideration when treating the Charcot foot. It is also important to note that certainly bisphosphonate treatment comes with its own risks, side effects and contraindications, which the clinician must take into account when considering this therapy.

CALCITONIN

Calcitonin is a polypeptide secreted from parafollicular C cells of the thyroid that can inhibit bone resorption by acting directly on osteoclast receptors. A common study that is referenced when considering calcitonin therapy in the treatment of the acute stage of the Charcot foot was performed by Bem and colleagues.[25] They performed a randomized controlled trial studying intranasal salmon calcitonin 200 IU daily in 32 patients with an acute Charcot foot. Both the calcitonin and the control group received calcium supplementation. To monitor disease progression, they measured skin temperature and bone metabolic turnover by measuring 1CTP and ALP. Nine patients had renal insufficiency, 5 in the calcitonin group and 4 in the control group. All patients were offloaded using removable contact cast or cast walkers. They found significant reduction in bone metabolic markers 1CTP and ALP during the first 3 months in the calcitonin group. No significant difference was seen with ALP concentration between groups at 6 months. There was no significant difference between groups in regards to temperature reduction. The authors concluded that calcitonin administration can reduce bone resorption in acute Charcot and is a reasonable option in patients with renal insufficiency. However, it would be beneficial for future studies to examine the long-term effects on patients who have received calcitonin therapy in the acute phase of Charcot and if this affected rates of limb salvage.

MONOCLONAL ANTIBODIES

As RANKL plays an important role in osteoclast regulation, denosumab, a fully human monoclonal antibody that targets RANKL, has been studied with its effects toward the treatment of the Charcot foot in the acute stage. Busch-Westbroek and colleagues[26] performed an observational study in 22 patients studying the efficacy of denosumab in the treatment of a Charcot foot. All patients had offloading measures with a TCC while also receiving calcium and vitamin D supplementation. They found that fracture resolution time was lower among the denosumab group. They also observed that time to clinical cessation of acute Charcot including time spent in the TCC, as well as malalignment of the Chopart-Lisfranc joint was significantly less in the denosumab group. At 12 month follow-up, the denosumab group had no Charcot events in the contralateral limb compared with 18% in the control group. There was also no amputations in the denosumab group at 12 months, whereas 3 patients in the control group underwent some level of amputation (1 TMA and 2 BKA) in 27% of patients. There was no significant difference between groups in regards to wound recurrence. It is noteworthy that 5 out of 11 patients in the control group used Alendronate, thus diminishing the quality of the control group. Although this study has its limitations, it does report the positive effects of denosumab on limb salvage and illustrates that patients had shorter time spent in the TCC in the acute stage with less deformity noted at the Chopart-Lisfranc joints. Shofler and colleagues[27] performed a prospective pilot study evaluating 7 patients treated with denosumab in the acute stage of Charcot. All patients received appropriate offloading and immobilization measures and were followed regularly up to 12 months. Although they did not have a control group, their average time for skin temperature to normalize, which also reflected time spent in a TCC, was 52 ± 17.89 days. This was significantly shorter time than was reported in Busch-Westbroek's study,[26] although they still used the similar 60 mg one-time injection dosing of denosumab and offloading measures. The ALP values measured showed an increase until week 4, then a decreasing trend from weeks 4 to 12, with a final gradual increase toward baseline at 12 months. They did trend inflammatory markers such as C-reactive protein (CRP) and erythrocyte sedimentation rate (ESR) and noted that they did not correspond to clinical activity. Although these studies show potential benefits of denosumab therapy in treatment of the acute Charcot foot with encouraging results, further high-level randomized controlled trials with longer term follow-up are warranted.

Other metabolic factors that affect bone resorption including calcium and vitamin D levels must be considered as well. It has been shown that diabetic patients who have low vitamin D levels leads to poor mineralization of bone.[28] Moreover, lower calcium levels can stimulate parathyroid hormone, which leads to increased bone resorption and eventual osteopenia.[29] Thus, it is important to monitor calcium and vitamin D levels and supplement as necessary in patients who present with an acute Charcot foot.

Although pharmacologic therapy for the treatment of the Charcot foot in the acute stage may show some short-term benefits, the literature and quality of evidence regarding this topic is rather weak with lack of long-term follow-up and strong comparisons.[30] Currently, it is not warranted to treat patients with an acute Charcot foot with antiresorptive or anti-inflammatory therapy until higher level evidence exists.[31] If the clinician does elect to treat with these agents, it is important that they are used in conjunction with nonweight-bearing and immobilization. Care must also be taken to evaluate all potential risks and side effects of these medications and how they apply on an individual patient basis. These antiresorptive and anti-inflammatory agents do not replace the mainstay of the treatment of the Charcot foot in the acute stage consisting of nonweight-bearing and immobilization of the affected lower extremity.

SUMMARY

The acute Charcot foot is a diagnostically difficult entity for clinicians. There should be a high level of clinical suspicion when a neuropathic patient presents with erythema, edema, and warmth of the foot or ankle. A thorough work-up should be done to rule out other causes. Radiographs can help rule out trauma and may show subtle changes of the involved joints initially. Venous duplex ultrasound can be used to rule out DVT, and MRI can be considered to rule out abscess or osteomyelitis, although an indium 111-WBC-labeled bone scan or bone biopsy may be more useful to differentiate osteomyelitis versus Charcot. Laboratories may also be useful including erythrocyte sedimentation rate, C-reactive protein, uric acid, and CBC with differential.

Once the diagnosis of Charcot has been made, it is important to quickly initiate appropriate management. The current best evidence recommends immobilization and nonweight-bearing for the duration of the Charcot process until the consolidation phase has been reached. Although various pharmacologic treatments including bisphosphonates, calcitonin, and monoclonal antibodies have been investigated for their role in managing acute Charcot, the use of these medications is not currently recommended and further research is necessary. Calcium and vitamin D should be optimized in Charcot patients to help improve osseous consolidation of the affected bone. Diabetic patients should also be encouraged to appropriately manage their diabetes to help improve the healing process and improve the outcomes of any potentially necessary surgical interventions.

Time should also be taken to explain to patients why adherence to immobilization and offloading is so critical in the treatment of Charcot. Patients need to have an understanding of the consequences of noncompliance including nonbraceable deformity, ulceration and infection, need for major reconstructive surgery, and amputation.

CLINICS CARE POINTS

- A high index of clinical suspicion for Charcot neuroarthropathy is necessary when evaluating neuropathic patients.
- Podiatric physicians have the opportunity to educate patients on the signs and symptoms of Charcot, which may increase a patients likelihood of correct diagnosis if this occurs.
- It is appropriate to be cautious and quickly initiate non-weightbearing and immobilization in patients that may have Charcot.

REFERENCES

1. Sohn MW, Stuck RM, Pinzur M, et al. Lower-extremity amputation risk after Charcot arthropathy and diabetic foot ulcer. Diabetes Care 2010;33(1):98–100.
2. Nielson DL, Armstrong DG. The natural history of Charcot's neuroarthropathy. Clin Podiatr Med Surg 2008;1:53–62.
3. Frykberg RG, Belczyk R. Epidemiology of the charcot foot. Clin Podiatr Med Surg 2008;25(1):17–28.
4. Eichenholtz SN. Charcot joints. Springfield, IL, USA: Charles C. Thomas; 1966.
5. Shibata T, Tada K, Hashizume C. The results of arthrodesis of the ankle for leprotic neuroarthropathy. J Bone Joint Surg Am 1990;72:749–56.
6. Brodsky JW. The diabetic foot. In: Coughlin MJ, Mann RA, Saltzman CL, editors. Surgery of the foot and ankle. 8. St. Louis, MO, USA: Mosby; 2006.
7. Guven MF, Karabiber A, Kaynak G, et al. Conservative and surgical treatment of the chronic Charcot foot and ankle. Diabet Foot Ankle 2013;4:2117.

8. Pakarinen TK, Laine HJ, Maenpaa H, et al. Long-term outcome and quality of life in patients with Charcot foot. Foot Ankle Surg 2009;15(4):187–91.

9. Griffiths DA, Kaminski MA. Duration of total contact casting for resolution of acute Charcot foot: a retrospective cohort study. J Foot Ankle Res 2021;14:44.

10. Game FL, Catlow R, Jones GR, et al. Audit of acute Charcot's disease in the UK: the CDUK study. Diabetologia 2021;55(1):32–5.

11. Milne TE, Rogers JR, Kinnear EM, et al. Developing an evidence-based clinical pathway for the assessment, diagnosis, and management of acute Charcot Neuro-Arthropathy: a systematic review. J Foot Ankle Res 2013;6(1):30.

12. Cook JJ, Cook EA. Protected weight bearing during treatment of acute charcot neuroarthropathy: a case series. Foot Ankle Online J 2011;4(7):1.

13. Nube VL, McGill M, Molyneaux L, et al. From acute to chronic: monitoring the progress of charcot's arthropathy. J Am Podiatr Med Assoc 2002;92(7):384–9.

14. Jeffcoate W, Lima J, Nobrega L. The charcot foot. Diabet Med 2000;17:253.

15. Yousaf S, Dawe EJC, Saleh A, et al. The acute Charcot foot in diabetics: diagnosis and management. Foot & Ankle 2018;3:568–73.

16. Drake MT, Clarke BL, Khosla S. Bisphosphonates: mechanism of action and role in clinical practice. Mayo Clin Proc 2008;83(9):1032–45.

17. Mabilleau G, Petrova NL, Edmonds ME, et al. Increased osteoclastic activity in acute Charcot's osteoarthropathy: the role of receptor activator of nuclear factor-kappaB ligand. Diabetologia 2008;51:1035–40.

18. Baumhauer JF, O'Keefe RJ, Schon LC, et al. Cytokineinduced osteoclastic bone resorption in charcot arthropathy: an immunohistochemical study. Foot Ankle Int 2006;27:797–800.

19. Gough A, Abraha H, Li F, et al. Measurement of markers of osteoclast and osteoblast activity in patients with acute and chronic diabetic Charcot neuroarthropathy. Diabet Med 1997;14:527–31.

20. Selby PL, Young MJ, Boulton AJ. Bisphosphonates: a new treatment for diabetic Charcot neuroarthropathy? Diabet Med 1994;11:28–31.

21. Moreno M, Gratacós J, Casado E, et al. [Usefulness of pamidronate in the treatment of charcot's arthropathy]. Reumatol Clin 2007;3:257–61.

22. Jude EB, Selby PL, Burgess J, et al. Bisphosphonates in the treatment of Charcot neuroarthropathy: a double-blind randomised controlled trial. Diabetologia 2001; 44:2032–7.

23. Pitocco D, Ruotolo V, Caputo S, et al. Six-month treatment with alendronate in acute Charcot neuroarthropathy: a randomized controlled trial. Diabetes Care 2005;28:1214–5.

24. Pakarinen TK, Laine HJ, Mäenpää H, et al. The effect of zoledronic acid on the clinical resolution of Charcot neuroarthropathy: a pilot randomized controlled trial. Diabetes Care 2011;34:1514–6.

25. Bem R, Jirkovská A, Fejfarová V, et al. Intranasal calcitonin in the treatment of acute Charcot neuroosteoarthropathy: a randomized controlled trial. Diabetes Care 2006;29:1392–4.

26. Busch-Westbroek TE, Delpeut K, Balm R, et al. Effect of single dose of RANKL antibody treatment on acute charcot neuroosteoarthropathy of the foot. Diabetes Care 2018;41:e21–2.

27. Shofler D, Hamedani E, Seun J, et al. Investigating the use of denosumab in the treatment of acute charcot neuroarthropathy. J Foot Ankle Surg 2021;60(2): 354–7.

28. Blakytny R, Spraul M, Jude EB. Review: the diabetic bone: a cellular and molecular perspective. Int J Low Extrem Wounds 2011;10:16–32.

29. Kaynak G, Birsel O, Guven MF, et al. An overview of the Charcot foot pathophysiology. Diabet Foot Ankle 2013;4:21117.
30. Durgia H, Sahoo J, Kamalanathan S, et al. Role of bisphosphonates in the management of the acute Charcot foot. World J Diabetes 2018;9(7):115–26.
31. Rastogi A, Bhansali A, Jude EB. Efficacy of medical treatment for Charcot neuroarthropathy: a systematic review and meta-analysis of randomized controlled trials. Acta Diabetol 2021;58(6):687–96.

Surgical Optimization for Charcot Patients

Kelsey J. Millonig, DPM, MPH[a],*, Rachel Gerber, DPM[b]

KEYWORDS

- Charcot • Peripheral vascular disease • metabolic bone profile • hemoglobin A1c
- vitamin D • osteomyelitis

KEY POINTS

- Patients with Charcot Neuroarthopathy have multiple morbidities that make them a challenge pre and post-reconstruction.
- Partner with colleagues in endocrinology, vascular, nutrition, primary care, etc. These individuals are essential in being able to perform a successful reconstructive surgery.
- Optimizing patients prior to surgery takes time, effort, and patients; to have successful outcomes we need to have multiple visits with these patients prior to surgery and honestly describe best and worse case scenarios.

Abbreviations	
TSH	Thyroid Stimulating Hormone
PTH	Parathyroid Hormone
DM	Diabetes Mellitus
CRPPS	Charcot Reconstruction Preoperative Prognostic Score
PEDIS	Perfusion, Extent, Depth, Infection, Sensation

INTRODUCTION

Reconstruction of the Charcot foot and ankle demonstrates significant challenges to the foot and ankle surgeon. At present, there is limited clear consensus on the best approach for preoperative optimization. The primary aim of Charcot reconstructions is to limit the risk of ulceration by providing a stable plantigrade foot allowing ambulation. However, often with or without reconstructive treatment there is a significant risk of amputation. The reported limb salvage rates in this population have been variable. Although there is a presence of outcome-based research, the role of preoperative

[a] East Village Foot & Ankle Surgeons, 500 East Court Avenue, Suite 314, Des Moines, IA 50309, USA; [b] AMITA Health Saint Joseph Hospital Chicago, 2900 North Lake Shore Drive, Chicago, IL 60657, USA
* Corresponding author.
E-mail address: Kelsey.J.Millonig@gmail.com

Clin Podiatr Med Surg 39 (2022) 595–604
https://doi.org/10.1016/j.cpm.2022.05.006
0891-8422/22/© 2022 Elsevier Inc. All rights reserved.

podiatric.theclinics.com

optimization to provide the best success of limb salvage and prevention of amputation is still relatively understudied. Pinzur and colleagues reported data with preoperative considerations including large bone deformity, long-standing ulceration with concomitant infection, regional osteopenia, obesity, and immunocompromised states as risks to intervention. Eschler and colleagues identified high-risk criteria associated with Charcot reconstructions using the CRPPS scoring system.[1] The investigator identified a PEDIS score of <7 as associated with successful limb salvage. However, the optimization of modifiable factors was not discussed. The focus of this article is the discussion of modifiable risk factors associated with Charcot reconstruction for preoperative optimization. The remainder of this article is organized as follows.

Diabetes
  Hemoglobin A1C

Peripheral vascular disease

Tobacco Use

Chronic Kidney Disease

Obesity

Hypertension

Edema

Albumin/Prealbumin

Metabolic Bone Profile
  Vitamin D/Calcium
  Thyroid TSH, PTH
  Osteopenia

Infection
  Wound
  Osteomyelitis

Diabetes

The presence of diabetes itself is an increased risk for loss of limb. Nondiabetic patients with Charcot neuroarthropathy are still 15 times more likely to return to ambulation after reconstruction than diabetic patients with well controlled glucose levels.[2] It is important to educate patients regarding their risk because of the metabolic impact of diabetes systemically and therefore the importance of optimizing their glucose control. It is estimated that 0.1% to 7.5% of patients with diabetes develop Charcot neuroarthropathy.[3]

Hemoglobin A1C

Surgical site infections have been found to increase when patients have a hemoglobin A1C (HbA1c) $\geq$ 8%, so it is recommended to delay surgery until the HbA1c can be decreased below that level.[4] In addition to referrals to endocrinology for management, it would also be beneficial to consider referral for nutritional education as the long-term health of these patients mostly depends on their nutrition. There may be clinical scenarios where the level of the deformity with impending soft tissue compromise requires surgical reconstruction with an HbA1c greater than 8%. Postoperative glycemic control will also reduce complication rates.[5] Sadoskas and colleagues[5] found that patients with a serum glucose greater than 200 mg/dL have a significantly higher risk of surgical site infection.

Peripheral Vascular Disease

The prevalence of peripheral vascular disease (PVD) in patients with Charcot neuro-arthropathy has been heavily debated in the literature with ranges from 4% to 40% being recorded in the last 20 years.[4,6–12] In patients greater than 40 year old, the prevalence of peripheral arterial disease (PAD) is estimated to be twice as high in patients with diabetes mellitus (10%) compared with that of the nondiabetic patients (5%).[9] In addition, in the presence of a diabetic foot ulcer, the incidence of PAD is found to be 49%.[13]

It is imperative to understand that there is no definitive noninvasive method for diagnosing PAD in the diabetic population. Owing to diabetic individuals having calcification of vessels, ankle-brachial indexes (ABIs) are frequently falsely elevated. The best results for diagnosing PVD in diabetics have been found by combining ABI tests with the toe-brachial index (TBI) tests especially in patients with an ABI $\geq$ 1.3.[14–16] This is because of ABI having high specificity and the TBI with high sensitivity. Qualitative waveform analysis has also been found to be a highly sensitive screening method for PVD in individuals with diabetes.[15] Alternatively, an arterial duplex may be used in combination with ABIs or TBIs as a reference standard to allow for more definitive information and diagnosis regarding vascular status.[17]

Patients who had Charcot with diabetes, PVD, and critical limb ischemia were found to have significantly lower rates of limb preservation (59.1%) a year after balloon angioplasty. Conversely, patients with just DM and critical limb ischemia had a limb preservation rate of 92.7%.[18] The risk of lower extremity amputations in patients with Charcot and PVD continues to be a concern even after surgical reconstructions. PVD caused by a 2.012 times increase in likelihood of having delayed healing and increased the risk of major lower extremity amputation by 4.414 fold in individuals with Charcot.[10]

It is imperative that preoperatively patients are evaluated preoperatively with vascular analysis beyond clinical examination findings. Even in the setting of palpable pedal pulses, the authors suggest obtaining arterial studies. With abnormal findings, it is imperative to provide an appropriate referral for revascularization before elective surgery to increase success for limb preservation.

Tobacco Use

It is well established that tobacco use is a risk factor for impaired wound healing, infection, delayed fracture healing, and prolonged hospital stay. Complications can be reduced by 40% if tobacco cessation is completed perioperatively.[19] The ideal time frame for this has been described as cessation not later than 8 weeks before surgery.[20] In elective lower extremity orthopedic surgery, patients required to quit preoperatively, 48% maintained smoking cessation for at least 1 year postoperatively. Of those who relapsed, approximately half stated that they did not resume smoking until at least 3 months postoperatively. Therefore, this particular period may be an important time for intensified smoking cessation counseling.[19] The use of tobacco products has been commonly associated with PVD and wound healing complications even in nondiabetic individuals. Charcot patients who had a history of smoking were found to have 2.4 times higher odds of having PVD.[10] These same individuals had a significantly increased likelihood to have delayed healing than their nonsmoking counterparts.[10]

Chronic Kidney Disease

Valabhji and colleagues found that 30% of patients with Charcot neuroarthropathy had end-stage renal disease (ESRD).[21] Patients with renal disease (renal disease: ESRD and chronic kidney disease [CKD]) are 3.5 times more likely to have PVD and if on dialysis have a 10 times higher rate of amputation.[10,22] The risk of major lower extremity amputations is also statistically higher for patients with renal disease.[10] This is secondary to wound healing complications, inhibited osseous union, sepsis, and cardiovascular disease. Raspovic and colleagues found that diabetic patients with ESRD requiring dialysis and lower extremity complications were found to have increased higher creatinine levels, lower hemoglobin levels, lower albumin levels, and higher rates ofPAD.[23]

Obesity

There is an association that has been established between increased body mass index (BMI) and the occurrence of Charcot neuroarthropathy.[24] Once patients are diagnosed with Charcot neuroarthropathy, these higher values of BMI values are associated with a higher occurrence of amputations.[24] Although the effect of BMI has not been well studied in regard to its effect on Charcot reconstructions, the general mentality is higher BMIs may lead to increased complications. This has been supported by prior research on BMI and foot and ankle surgery. In a case series of 18 patients who underwent tibiocalcaneal arthrodesis, Love and colleagues found that patients were at an increased risk of postoperative complications if they had a BMI >25; these complications included nonunions, infections, and hardware failures.[25] Increased BMIs have been associated with decreased physical function after fixation of ankle fractures.[26] These studies may provide useful insight regarding the effect of BMI on patients undergoing reconstructive surgery for Charcot joints.

Hypertension

Hypertension has been found to be a statistically significant risk factor for delayed healing.[10] In addition, hypertension is a known independent risk factor for PAD.

Edema

Preoperative edema control is important to consider in prevention of wound healing complications postoperatively. In addition, consideration for edema is important if using an external fixator to ensure adequate space is left with ring fixation. Minimally invasive techniques for Charcot neuroarthropathy may be an optimal consideration for concern of edema.

Albumin/Prealbumin

Evaluating these laboratory results is important for consideration for protein markers of nutritional status for wound healing.[23] It is well established that preoperative hypoalbuminemia can impact wound healing. However, this is even more critical in the diabetic population. Cheng and colleagues found that patients with a diabetic foot infection with hypoalbuminemia (<3.5 g/dL) demonstrated a 2.5-fold higher risk of nonhealing at postoperative 28 days than patients with normal levels.[27] Therefore, preoperative serum albumin levels should be analyzed, optimized, and used as a biomarker for predicting postoperative healing.

Metabolic Bone Profile

Vitamin D/calcium

It is well understood that vitamin D is crucial for optimal arthrodesis. A 2017 study of patients undergoing elective foot and ankle surgery showed that patients with vitamin D deficiency insufficiency were 8.1 times more likely to develop a nonunion.[28] Diabetic patients both with and without Charcot neuroarthropathy have significantly lower vitamin D levels (serum 25-hydroxyvitamin D) than nondiabetic patients.[29] In addition, owing to the need for bioactivation of 25-hydroxyvitamin D3 in the kidney, patients with concomitant renal disease are more typically deficient and also more challenging to optimize as a result.

Thyroid levels

Thyroid hormones are essential for bone mass maintenance, and hypothyroidism yields impared bone formation. Suppression of thyroid stimulating hormone can have an increased risk for osteoporotic fracture.[30] For adult patients, T3 regulates bone turnover and bone mineral density (BMD). With abnormal thyroid levels, patients lose optimal bone strength, and population studies indicate that hypothyroidism and hyperthyroidism are associated with an increased risk of fracture. In addition, literature has also demonstrated that TSH may have direct actions in bone cells. The full discussion of the endocrine pathways that regulate bone mass is beyond the scope of this article. However, completing a metabolic bone laboratory analysis should be considered preoperatively as this may affect the success rate of the patient postoperatively.[31] Appropriate referral to endocrinology should be considered as necessary.

Osteopenia

Osteopenia has long been considered to be a classic finding of Charcot neuroarthropathy.[32] Charcot patients have commonly been found to have reduced BMD in their peripheral skeleton, but it is unknown if Charcot causes reduced BMD or if decreased BMD leads to Charcot.[33–36]

Subclassification of the pattern of injury in Charcot neuroarthropathy patients has found three subgroups: fracture, dislocation, and combination fracture–dislocation type patterns.[37] Individuals with fracture Charcot neuroarthropathy were found to have significantly lower t-scores (SD from site- and gender-matched healthy young adult means) and z-scores (SDs from age-, site-, and gender-matched means) than individuals with dislocation Charcot.[37] The distribution of the fracture patients' t-scores may be found in **Fig. 1**. Of the patients that had dislocation Charcot, only four individuals had t-scores less than −1.0.[37]

Infection

Wound/osteomyelitis

Owing to the deformities that occur with Charcot neuroarthropathy, patients are at increased risk of lower extremity ulcerations which commonly lead to infections and

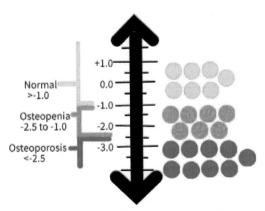

Fig. 1. Distribution of the fragmentation Charcot patients in Herbst and colleagues based on WHO criteria.[37,38]

Preoperative Charcot Reconstruction Checklist	Yes	No
1. Does the patient have diabetes?		
1a. If yes what was the last HbA1c?		
2. Does the patient have known clinical signs of PVD?		
2a. Recommend ordering ABI, TBI, and/or arterial duplex regardless of clinical findings		
3. Does the patient have any history of Tobacco use?		
3a. If yes recommend smoking cessation for minimum of 8 weeks preop to 3 months postop and completing 2a.		
4. Does the patient have Chronic Kidney Disease?		
4a. If yes recommend completing 2a.		
5. What is the patients BMI?		
6. Does the patient have Hypertension?		
6a. If yes recommend completing 2a and advising patient of possible wound healing complications		
7. Does the patient have Edema?		
7a. If yes consider treatment for edema control and minimally invasive technqiues		
8. What is the patients preoperative albumin/prealbumin?		
9. Is the patient Vitamin D deficient?		
9a. If yes consider optimizing patient prior to surgery		
10. What was the patients preoperative TSH and T3 level?		
10a. If abnormal consider sending patient to endocrinology for optimization prior to surgery		
11. Does the patient have known osteopenia?		
11a. Regardless of answer to 11, What was the patients most recent t-score/z-score?		
12. Does the patient have an ulceration?		
12a. If yes, obtain deep tissue cultures		
12b. Is there a soft tissue infection?		
12c. Is there any chance of bony involvement?		
If yes obtain bone biopsy		
12d. Is there osteomyelitis present?		

Fig. 2. Example of preoperative optimization checklist.

osteomyelitis. Foot ulcers have been reported to occur in 11% to 60% of all diabetics with Charcot deformity.[39–42] In diabetics, 50% to 60% of ulcers become infected.[43] The previous research has shown that osteomyelitis occurs in 20% of patients who experience an ulceration is more likely to occur in larger and deeper ulcerations and may be present in greater than 60% of infected diabetic foot ulcers.[44–48]

Individuals 65+ years of age with ulcerations are 13 times more likely to have a major lower extremity amputation than their age-matched nonulcerated counterparts.[49] However, age is not a large factor in the equation as individuals less than 65 years of age with an ulcer were 12 times more likely to have an amputation.[49]

Many physicians prefer to heal the ulcer before reconstructive surgery.[50–52]

In cases where resolution of the ulcer before correction is not possible, deep cultures and bone biopsies should be taken before reconstructive surgery to rule out soft tissue infection and osteomyelitis. Numerous authors have been able to perform reconstructive surgery and heal the ulcer simultaneously. Acute deformity correction has been used successfully to heal and prevent recurrence of ulceration.[53] Wrotslavsky and colleagues found using gradual correction can safely and accurately correct the Meary and calcaneal inclination angles while also healing 100% of ulcers.[54] In addition, a staged procedure with the management of ulceration or osteomyelitis with antibiotic spacer and/or masquelet technique if needed can be used.

SUMMARY

As demonstrated in this article, there are several factors that impact the success of Charcot neuroarthropathy surgical reconstruction beyond the surgical technique. It is imperative that physicians consider the factors described above for surgical optimization preoperatively (**Fig. 2**).

DISCLOSURE

K.J. Millonig is a Consultant for Orthofix.

REFERENCES

1. Eschler A, Gradl G, Wussow A, et al. Prediction of complications in a high-risk cohort of patients undergoing corrective arthrodesis of late stage Charcot deformity based on the PEDIS score. BMC Musculoskelet Disord 2015;16:349.

2. Cates NK, Wagler EC, Bunka TJ, et al. Charcot reconstruction: outcomes in patients with and without diabetes. J Foot Ankle Surg 2020;59(6):1229–33.

3. Frykberg Robert G, Belczyk Ronald. Epidemiology of the charcot foot. Clin Podiatric Med Surg 2008;25(1):17–28.

4. Wukich DK, Crim BE, Frykberg RG, et al. Neuropathy and poorly controlled diabetes increase the rate of surgical site infection after foot and ankle surgery. J Bone Joint Surg Am 2014;96(10):832–9.

5. Sadoskas D, Suder NC, Wukich DK. Perioperative glycemic control and the effect on surgical site infections in diabetic patients undergoing foot and ankle surgery. Foot Ankle Spec 2016;9(1):24–30.

6. Chantelau E. The perils of procrastination: effects of early vs. delayed detection and treatment of incipient Charcot fracture. Diabet Med 2005;22(12):1707e12.

7. Sohn MW, Lee TA, Stuck RM, et al. Mortality risk of Charcot arthropathy compared with that of diabetic foot ulcer and diabetes alone. Diabetes Care 2009;32(5):816e21.

8. Salini D, Harish K, Minnie P, et al. Prevalence of Charcot Arthropathy in Type 2 Diabetes Patients Aged over 50 Years with Severe Peripheral Neuropathy: A Retrospective Study in a Tertiary Care South Indian Hospital. Indian J Endocrinol Metab 2018;22(1):107–11.

9. Gregg Ew, Sorlie P, Paulos-Ram R, et al. Prevalence of lower-extremity disease in the US adult population >= 40 years of age with and without diabetes. Diabetes Care 2004;27:1591–7.

10. Cates NK, Elmarsafi T, Akbari CM, et al. Complications of charcot reconstruction in patients with peripheral arterial disease. J Foot Ankle Surg 2021;60(5):941–5. Epub 2021 Apr 1.

11. Cates NK, Elmarsafi T, Bunka TJ, et al. Peripheral vascular disease diagnostic related outcomes in diabetic charcot reconstruction. J Foot Ankle Surg 2019; 58(6):1058–63.

12. Wukich DK, Raspovic KM, Suder NC. Prevalence of peripheral arterial disease in patients with diabetic Charcot c. J Foot Ankle Surg 2016;55(4):727–31.

13. Prompers L, Huijberts M, Apelqvist J, et al. High prevalence of ischaemia, infection and serious comorbidity in patients with diabetic foot disease in Europe. Baseline results from the Eurodiale study. Diabetologia 2007;50:18–25.

14. Wukich DK, Shen W, Raspovic KM, et al. Noninvasive arterial testing in patients with diabetes: a guide for foot and ankle surgeons. Foot Ankle Int 2015;36(12): 1391–9.

15. Williams DT, Harding KG, Price P. An evaluation of the efficacy of methods used in screening for lower-limb arterial disease in diabetes. Diabetes Care 2005;28(9): 2206–10.

16. Brooks B, Dean R, Patel S, et al. TBI or not TBI: that is the question. Is it better to measure toe pressure than ankle pressure in diabetic patients? Diabet Med 2001; 18(7):528–32.

17. Crawford F, Welch K, Andras A, et al. Ankle brachial index for the diagnosis of lower limb peripheral arterial disease. Cochrane Database Syst Rev 2016;9(9): CD010680. Published 2016 Sep 14.

18. Çildağ MB, Köseoğlu ÖFK. The effect of charcot neuroarthropathy on limb preservation in diabetic patients with foot wound and critical limb ischemia after balloon angioplasty. J Diabetes Res 2017;2017:5670984. Epub 2017 Aug 29.

19. Smith DH, McTague MF, Weaver MJ, et al. Durability of smoking cessation for elective lower extremity orthopaedic surgery. J Am Acad Orthop Surg 2019; 27(16):613–20.

20. Myers K, Hajek P, Hinds C, et al. Stopping smoking shortly before surgery and postoperative complications: a systematic review and meta-analysis. Arch Intern Med 2011;171(11):983–9. Epub 2011 Mar 14.

21. Valabhji J. Foot problems in patients with diabetes and chronic kidney disease. J Ren Care 2012;38(Suppl 1):99–108. PMID: 22348369.

22. Ndip A, Rutter MK, Vileikyte L, et al. Dialysis treatment is an independent risk factor for foot ulceration in patients with diabetes and stage 4 or 5 chronic kidney disease. Diabetes Care 2010;33:1811–6.

23. Raspovic KM, Ahn J, La Fontaine J, et al. End-stage renal disease negatively affects physical quality of life in patients with diabetic foot complications. Int J Low Extrem Wounds 2017;16(2):135–42. Epub 2017 May 4.

24. Bandeira MA, Dos Santos ALG, Woo K, et al. Incidence and predictive factors for amputations derived from charcot's neuroarthropathy in persons with diabetes. Int J Low Extrem Wounds 2021. https://doi.org/10.1177/15347346211025893. Epub ahead of print.

25. Love B, Alexander B, Ray J, et al. Outcomes of tibiocalcaneal arthrodesis in high-risk patients: an institutional cohort of 18 patients. Indian J Orthop 2020;54(1): 14–21.

26. Dean Daniel M, Ho Bryant S, Lin Albert, et al. Predictors of patient-reported function and pain outcomes in operative ankle fractures. Foot Ankle Int 2017;38(5): 496–501.
27. Cheng P, Dong Y, Hu Z, et al. Biomarker prediction of postoperative healing of diabetic foot ulcers: a retrospective observational study of serum albumin. J Wound Ostomy Continence Nurs 2021;48(4):339–44.
28. Moore KR, Howell MA, Saltrick KR, et al. Risk factors associated with nonunion after elective foot and ankle reconstruction: a case-control study. J Foot Ankle Surg 2017;56(3):457–62.
29. Yoho RM, Frerichs J, Dodson NB, et al. A comparison of vitamin D levels in nondiabetic and diabetic patient populations. J Am Podiatr Med Assoc 2009;99(1):35–41.
30. Galliford TM, Murphy E, Williams AJ, et al. Effects of thyroid status on bone metabolism: a primary role for thyroid stimulating hormone or thyroid hormone? Minerva Endocrinol 2005;30(4):237–46.
31. Williams GR. Actions of thyroid hormones in bone. Endokrynol Pol 2009;60(5): 380–8.
32. Purewal T. Charcot's diabetic neuroarthropathy: pathogenesis, diagnosis and management. Pract Diabetes Int 1996;13:88–91.
33. Childs M, Armstrong DG, Edelson GW. Is Charcot arthropathy a late sequela of osteoporosis in patients with diabetes mellitus? J Foot Ankle Surg 1998;37:437–9.
34. Young MJ, Marshall A, Adams JE, et al. Osteopenia, neurological dysfunction, and the development of Charcot neuroarthropathy. Diabetes Care 1995;18:34–8.
35. Cundy TF, Edmonds ME, Watkins PJ. Osteopenia and metatarsal fractures in diabetic neuropathy. Diabet Med 1985;2:461–4.
36. Jirkovska AP, Kasalicky P, Boucek P, et al. Calcaneal ultrasonomentry in patients with Charcot osteoarthropathy and its relationship with densitometry in the lumbar spine and femoral neck and with markers of bone turnover. Diabet Med 2001;18: 495–500.
37. Herbst SA, Jones KB, Saltzman CL. Pattern of diabetic neuropathic arthropathy associated with the peripheral bone mineral density. J Bone Joint Surg Br 2004;86:378–83.
38. Kanis JA. Assessment of fracture risk and its application to screening for postmenopausal osteoporosis: synopsis of a WHO report. WHO Study Group. Osteoporos Int 1994;4:368–81.
39. Pakarinen TK, Laine HJ, Mäenpää H, et al. Long-term outcome and quality of life in patients with Charcot foot. Foot Ankle Surg 2009;15(4):187–91.
40. Leung HB, Ho YC, Wong WC. Charcot foot in a Hong Kong Chinese diabetic population. Hong Kong Med J 2009;15(3):191–5.
41. Fabrin J, Larsen K, Holstein PE. Long-term follow-up in diabetic Charcot feet with spontaneous onset. Diabetes Care 2000;23(6):796–800.
42. Armstrong DG, Todd WF, Lavery LA, et al. The natural history of acute Charcot's arthropathy in a diabetic foot specialty clinic. Diabet Med 1997;14(5):357–63.
43. Armstrong DG, Boulton AJM, Bus SA. Diabetic foot ulcers and their recurrence. N Engl J Med 2017;376:2367e2375.
44. Kagna O, Srour S, Melamed E, et al. 18F-FDG PET/CT imaging in the diagnosis of the osteomyelitis in the diabetic foot. Eur J Med Mol Imaging 2012;39:1545–50.
45. Lavery LA, Armstrong DG, Wunderlich RP, et al. Risk factors for foot infections in individuals with diabetes. Diabetes Care 2006;29(6):1288e1293.
46. Lipsky BA. Osteomyelitis of the foot in diabetic patients. Clin Infect Dis 1997;25: 1318–26.

47. Wrobel JS, Connolly JE. Making the diagnosis of osteomyelitis. The role of prevalence. J Am Podiatr Med Assoc 1998;88:337–43.
48. Norden CW. Acute and chronic osteomyelitis. Infect Dis 1999;2:43–8.
49. Sohn MW, Stuck RM, Pinzur M, et al. Lower-extremity ampu- tation risk after Charcot arthropathy and diabetic foot ulcer. Diabetes Care 2010;33(1):98–100.
50. Clohisy DR, Thompson RC Jr. Fractures associated with neuropathic arthropathy in adults who have juvenile-onset diabetes. J Bone Joint Surg Am 1988;70:1192–200.
51. Sammarco GJ, Conti SF. Surgical treatment of neuroarthropathic foot deformity. Foot Ankle Int 1998;19:102–9.
52. Sammarco VJ, Sammarco GJ, Walker EW Jr, et al. Midtarsal arthrodesis in the treatment of Charcot arthropathy. J Bone Joint Surg Am 2009;91:80–91.
53. Mittlmeier T, Klaue K, Haar P, et al. Should one consider primary surgical reconstruction in charcot arthropathy of the feet? Clin Orthop Relat Res 2010;468(4):1002–11.
54. Wrotslavsky P, Kriger SJ, Hammer-Nahman SM, et al. Computer-assisted gradual correction of Charcot foot deformities: an in-depth evaluation of stage one of a planned two-stage approach to Charcot Reconstruction. J Foot Ankle Surg 2020;59(4):841–8.

Beaming the Charcot Foot

William Grant, DPM, MS, FACFAS*, Lisa Grant-McDonald, DPM, AACFAS

KEYWORDS

- Beaming • Charcot neuroarthropathy • Truss

KEY POINTS

- Beaming is a method to simultaneously anatomically realign and reinforce the pathologic Charcot diabetic foot.
- Charcot-specific implants are now available, some of which may, through their inherent properties, enhance the durability of the correction.
- The use of truss/tie rod principle used in carpentry and the engineering arts may enhance the durability of correction.

In 2021 there are 34.2 million Americans living with diabetes, and nearly 0.08%-7.5% will suffer from Charcot Neuroarthropathy.[1] Since Banting and Best's 1923 breakthrough discovery of insulin, diabetics have continuously lived longer thanks to advances in medical science.[2,3] Sadly, living longer does not always translate into living well. Diabetics are beset by complications to virtually every organ system secondary to their underlying metabolic disorder. The "organ" of locomotion is not spared, and diabetics have multiple pedal issues including peripheral vascular disease, sensory and autonomic neuropathy, and metabolic bone disease.[4] One of the most devastating disorders this population faces is diabetic Charcot arthropathy. This destructive multi factorial process acts on bone and ligament alike producing seemingly random structural disfigurement of the foot and attendant ulcers; many of which are not treatable by standard wound care methods.

The Charcot foot can be surgically repaired; however, at this time, outcomes are not clearly predictable, leading some practitioners to assume that bracing is the most reliable treatment. The goal of surgical correction is to create a stable and plantigrade foot, free of significant risk of recurrent breakdown, collapse, or ulceration. Until recently, only patients who were unbraceable, acutely infected, or ulcerated were recommended for surgery. Amputation below the knee remains a clear option for the Charcot patient population. Studies addressing quality of life (QOL) in Charcot patients identify a significant impact on this population, labeling their health outlook as worse than those with end-stage renal disease and some cancers.[5-8] Evidence suggests that patient QOL improves the following reconstruction. A return to walkability and function

Tidewater Foot and Ankle, 760 Independence Boulevard, Virginia Beach, VA 23455, USA
* Corresponding author.
E-mail address: charcotking@yahoo.com

Clin Podiatr Med Surg 39 (2022) 605–627
https://doi.org/10.1016/j.cpm.2022.05.007
0891-8422/22/© 2022 Elsevier Inc. All rights reserved.
podiatric.theclinics.com

has been noted in reconstruction patients as well, furthering the interest in attempted limb salvage. A new study by Albright and colleagues examined the cost-effectiveness and quality-adjusted life years (QALY) of surgical reconstruction as compared with lifetime bracing and trans-tibial amputation.[9] In this analysis, they found Charcot patients without foot ulcers or with infected foot ulcers who underwent reconstruction improved the QALYs and showed reasonable cost-effectiveness when compared with lifetime bracing. This suggests that early intervention on Charcot foot is favored over lifetime bracing.

Methods of surgical correction in the Charcot midfoot are not clearly defined. At present, there are no available studies that have established the superiority of any fixation construct. Numerous constructs have been described to address midfoot fracture and dislocation.[10–12] Few, however, have been proven to demonstrate long-term benefit. Many experienced surgeons use locking plates, which are commonly used in foot and ankle reconstructive surgery. This familiarity likely predicts their use in Charcot repair. The early failures of the plate and screw construct led surgeons to refocus on the limitations of hardware. Their work has been published and demonstrates a strong consideration regarding hardware to address the deformity. Sammarco first mentioned the term "super constructs" in 2009,[13] this appellation has gained favor in the peer-review press (**Fig. 1**). A super construct was established as a method to extend the area of fixation past the area of disorder in hopes of gaining material strength. Many surgeons hoped that by lengthening their areas of fixation, stability would preclude failure. Unfortunately, the use of a super construct does not seem to mitigate the risk of hardware failure; however, it is still considered an essential principle in the reconstruction of the Charcot foot.

An alternative to the use of plates and interfragmentary screws is a technique known as beaming. First described in the mid-1990's, beaming was a method used to stabilize Charcot foot through the use of intramedullary fixation.[14] Generally, beaming can be described as the placement of large diameter screws either cannulated or solid (often referred to as bolts) down the medullary canals of one or more ray segments.[14,15] The medial column beam is started in the first metatarsal head and extends into the bone of the midtarsal joints, thus producing a "super construct" (**Fig. 2**). The linear, intramedullary screw aligns the deranged bone segments into a facsimile of a normally shaped foot in all 3 body planes. Additionally, as the Charcot

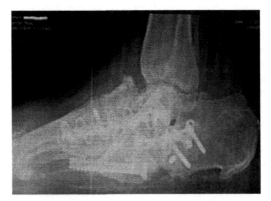

Fig. 1. An example of a "Superconstruct" that is meant to fixate past the area of involvement. A combination of locking plates and large diameter orthopedic screws has been placed to stabilize the Charcot foot.

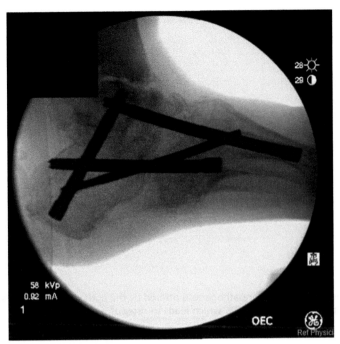

Fig. 2. An example of midfoot beaming. This super construct incorporates joints, which were uninvolved in this patient during the initial collapse pattern.

bone is abnormal, the large size screw gives structural support to the foot, which we will address in greater detail.

MECHANICS OF BEAMING

The pathophysiology of Charcot foot has yet to be fully described. A unifying theory of pathophysiology has yet to be elucidated. Numerous metabolic pathways have been described to evidence the derangements seen in the bone and ligament, but further research is required to substantiate these theories (**Fig. 3**).[16–20] It is well understood that the mechanical properties of the resultant damaged bone are abnormal, lacking the cellularity and mechanical strength of normal bone. La Fontaine and colleagues identified significant abnormality of Charcot bone, showing its immature/woven state and inability to appropriately mineralize.[21] Unlike other methods of fixation, beaming was designed to combat the limitations of Charcot bone. The placement of intramedullary devices obviates the need for healthy bone. The beam instead acts as a load share with the bone, placing no additional requirements on the site of union. Additionally, the beams allow for the extension of load sharing along the entirety of the medial and lateral column, or the creation of a "superconstruct."

To understand the challenges associated with reinforcing insufficient Charcot bone, a few fundamental engineering principles should be presented. During mid-stance position, the weight of the body loads along the foot and distributes over the parts of the foot that bare weight. For simplicity, let's assume the heel and the medial column of the foot are solely baring the weight of the body. As the weight is shared across the leaver arm, the weight creates a bending moment at every point along the medial column. A bending moment is a rotational force that occurs when a force is applied

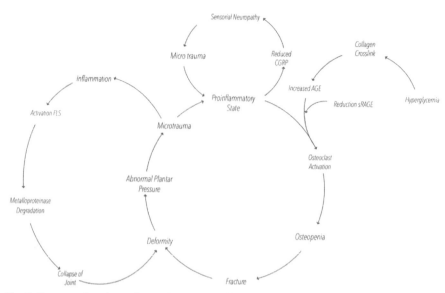

Fig. 3. Suggested pathway for pathogenesis offered by the authors. The cycle is largely propelled by a proinflammatory state, which leads to osseous destruction.

perpendicularly to a point (x) at a given distance away from that point (y). In our example, a bending moment can be calculated between any fixed points along the medial column and is used to identify the rotational force generated along that leaver arm. The bending moment may be used to explain the forces impacting joint interfaces or the hardware that lies along that moment arm. Bending moment is calculated as the perpendicular force multiplied by the distance from the load-bearing area. Because the bending moment is simply the bend that occurs in a beam due to a moment, bending moments can be calculated to determine the diameter of a beam needed to reinforce a given weight/load. Additionally, material strength of the beam, or whether or not the beam can be cannulated, can also be calculated. With the appropriate formulas, a safety factor can be calculated, so that episodes of overload do not result in immediate beam failure. **Fig. 4** demonstrates a beam running from the metatarsal head through the talus. As the metatarsal head is whereby the weight is absorbed (as well as the heel), there is a moment created along the shaft of the beam. Because the calculation of moment force is identified as force over distance, the joint furthest from the metatarsal head will "see" the largest moment force. The talonavicular joint is the joint, which receives the greatest moment. Not surprisingly, this anatomic location is often times the point of beam failure.

Using the above calculation we find that a beam made of surgical stainless steel, with a 7.4 mm outer diameter and a 2.8 mm cannulation provides a two times safety factor for a 300-pound person in the static stance position. Interestingly, the calculations show that a solid beam of the same material would need to be approximately 7.1 mm in diameter for the same safety factor. As such, the difference in diameter is not great enough to introduce the complexity of placing a solid beam in Charcot reconstruction. The engineering principles of beaming are the same that are used in the construction of buildings. Given the insufficiency in starting material (Charcot bone), a beam can be applied to stabilize the columns of the foot for pedal propulsion. Beaming is an engineering answer to a metabolic disorder and has been developed to

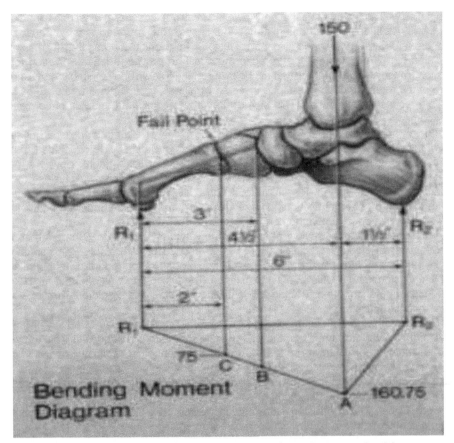

Fig. 4. The bending moment can be calculated with a force diagram. Point (B) represents the segment of the Lisfranc joint and is 37in/lbs. of bending moment force. This can be used to solve for the correct diameter of a beam.

specifically address the limitations of pedal architecture. With the advent of new Charcot-specific hardware, the principles of beaming have been improved to protect against hardware failure and subsequent reoccurrence of deformity.

Beaming in the Literature

Nearly 25 years after beaming was first described, an increasing body of literature, mostly level 4, has addressed the validity of this procedure. Early failures were identified with insufficient Charcot-specific hardware in which Wiewiorski and Yasui reported on the use of solid 6.5 mm bolts for Charcot midfoot.[22] Follow-up at 27 months reported no beam breakage; however, 3 out of 8 cases showed a significant migration of the bolt and required removal. There were no cases of reulceration and anatomic correction was mostly preserved, but hardware loosening was a concern.

Butt and colleagues who reported on a consecutive series of bolt failures performed further investigation into early beam failure.[23] These surgeons reported on 10 feet (9 patients) that they attempted to fuse the medial column using a 6.0 mm solid bolt. It should be noted that 6 of the cases also underwent hindfoot fusion with a retrograde nail. Results included significant improvement of the talo-metatarsal angle (Meary's angle) as well as the calcaneal pitch. However, in all but 2 cases, at least one joint did not fuse. Additionally, the bone migrated in 6 cases. They reported that 4 of those 6 cases were revised with good evidence of fusion. Their conclusion was that the medial column bolt is satisfactory for correction, but fails to provide adequate fixation for fusion. These authors suggest that the bolt was unacceptable and resulted in early failure of the reconstruction.[10] Despite these early failures, beaming still was used as a viable reconstructive option. This paved the way later for meta-analysis of surgical outcomes.

Lowery and colleagues completed a systematic review of all articles published in the world literature from 1963 to 2009 on Charcot reconstruction.[24] He concluded that arthrodesis was only used after the failure of conservative treatment. However, of the 246 patients undergoing arthrodesis, 76.4% showed complete fusion and 22.4% incomplete fusion. His study found an 80%–100% minor complication rate with the use of external fixation.[6] The results from this analysis supported beaming as an effective construct in the correction of Charcot midfoot.

In another systematic review of surgical interventions for Charcot, Shazadeh and colleagues reviewed 9 articles between 2006 and 2016, with a follow-up ranging from 12 to 63 months.[25] They found the most common fixation reported were medial column fusions and multilevel external fixation. The fusion rate was reported as 91% and the amputation rate as 6%, again identifying beaming as a predictable and effective reconstructive technique.[7]

Schneekloth and colleagues reported on a total of 860 patients operated on for Charcot neuroarthropathy.[26] Of these, 116 were for midfoot arthrodesis. They found no ideal timing for Charcot repair based on the Eichenholtz Classification, and in a 54-year review from 1960 to 2014, found that midfoot Charcot was the most common site for surgery. They reported that no significant data from that review favored external fixation or internal fixation.[8]

Ford, Cohen, Davis, and Jones reported clinical outcomes of Charcot patients with midfoot osteotomy and stabilization with intramedullary nails.[27] Their cohort was taken from patients treated between January 2013 and July 2016. Minimum follow-up to be included was 1 year and 25 patients met the criterion for inclusion. They found at 1-year follow-up, 84% of this group demonstrated an ulcer-free, stable plantigrade foot. Overall, however, only 46% of patients studied demonstrated united midfoot osteotomies, at 18 months postoperatively. Approximately 24% of their group developed a deep infection, and all had a history of ulceration before surgery. Four patients, 16%, progressed to a major amputation, all with a prior history of deep infection and ulceration. They concluded that while most patients met the criteria of an ulcer-free plantigrade foot postoperatively, the complication rate was high, especially among those with a history of ulceration.

Cates and colleagues recently writing in the Journal of Foot and Ankle Surgery, looked at postoperative outcomes of surgery of the Charcot foot. Specifically, they questioned if there was a difference in outcomes between Charcot dislocations versus Charcot fractures of the foot.[28] Secondarily, they investigated a similar difference with combination fracture-dislocation patients. Fascinatingly, dislocation patients had a statistically significantly higher rate of broken hardware and ostectomy revision surgery compared with pure fracture. Charcot dislocation pattern was 12 times more likely to require ostectomy and 8 times more likely to have osteomyelitis compared with Charcot fracture-dislocation patterns. Patients with a pure fracture pattern were 58.8 times more likely to have a talonavicular joint breakdown.

The dislocation pattern demonstrated a higher propensity for residual collapse, as evidenced by broken hardware, osteomyelitis, and revisional ostectomy.[9] The results from this study addressed the concerns for revision and reoccurrence of deformity and a potential risk factor to explain these findings.

Richter and colleagues reported on 48 feet (47 patients) from three centers in Germany.[29] The diagnosis was diabetic Charcot in 80.1%. All underwent reconstruction with a "Medial Fusion Bolt." They reported wound-healing problems in 21% of their cohort. 13% experienced reulceration. 6% required reoperation for loss of correction, and their union rate was 98% at final follow-up. Two patients require a trans-tibial amputation for deep infection and 3 "minor" foot amputations. Failure was more frequent when only one bolt was used compared with when 2 or 3 were used, and no gastrocnemius recession was performed. Their conclusions were that the Medial Fusion Bolt was a valuable tool for Charcot foot, with minimal loss of correction and high union rates. The use of a minimum of 2 bolts was recommended to avoid recurrent deformity.

A recent report compared the currently available Charcot-specific implants for beaming. Four-point bending tests evaluated each implant for flexural strength.[30] Cantilever bending tests placed maximum bending moments on the main thread of the implant to assess thread strength. Thread pullout tested the various implants by fixing the implant into a saw-bone block on a platform, with the opposite end connected to a loading actuator. The 7.4 mm cannulated stainless steel beam was superior to a 7.0 cannulated titanium beam and a 6.5 mm solid titanium bolt on all measures. When smaller Charcot-specific implants were tested in the same manner, the 5.4 mm cannulated stainless steel screw demonstrated higher stiffness, force to failure, tip fatigue strength, and thread pullout strength than a 5.0 mm solid titanium bolt.

They simply concluded that greater stiffness would resist deformation and improve stability. Greater static failure load and fatigue limit improve the implant's ability to withstand higher, repetitive loads before it fails. Although this study was a corporate-funded study, the report does identify some key mechanical requirements to avoid hardware failure.

Beaming Technique for Charcot Midfoot Reconstruction

The principles and actual practice of beaming the columns are best explained with visual examples. The pictures provided depict a salvage of an unstable Charcot diabetic foot occurring in a 74-year-old patient with a history of diabetes mellitus, peripheral neuropathy, peripheral vascular disease, and coronary artery disease (CAD).

The patient presented to the office for physical examination and radiographs before surgical intervention (**Fig. 5**). The radiographs reveal a negative Meary's angle in a sagittal view and divergent Meary's angle in the transverse view. Again, the lateral radiograph shows a negative calcaneal inclination angle with the abnormal alignment of the cuboid, which seems plantar prominent. The medial cuneiform has displaced medially, with a homolateral dislocation of the Lisfranc joint, and there is faulting of the talonavicular joint. These radiographic findings translate into a clinical picture of ulceration beneath the cuboid and distortion of the longitudinal arch, with rocker bottom appearance (**Fig. 6**). Following a comprehensive preoperative workup, the patient was taken to the operating theater for definitive acute correction of the Charcot deformity.

ACHILLES TENDON LENGTHENING

The Achilles tendon should be formally lengthened in virtually all Charcot diabetic midfoot reconstructions. Gastrocnemius recession is, in the authors' opinion, insufficient to address the posterior compartment contracture. The peer-review literature supports the presence of glycosylation of the tendon with attendant contracture, which

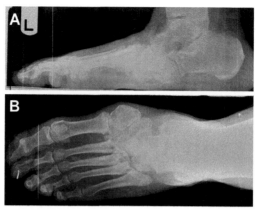

Fig. 5. 54-year-old man with Charcot Midfoot fracture dislocation. **(Fig. 5**B) Anterior/Posterior projection demonstrates a homolateral dislocation of Tarsometatarsal joint and midtarsal subluxation. **(Fig. 5**A)Lateral projection indicated a negative calcaneal inclination (-2°), and Talonavicular faulting with negative Meary's angle of (-5°).

is profound and worsens the collapse of the midfoot.[31,32] Additionally, Achilles contracture produces negative calcaneal inclination angles allowing increased forefoot stress. Increased bending force through the midtarsal joints increases the likelihood of hardware failure and reoccurrence of deformity.

Open tendo-Achilles lengthening (TAL) commences with a 6-cm incision placed medial to the border of the mid-substance of the tendon and extending 3 to 4 cm above the insertion **(Fig. 7)**. The tendon is gently brought out of the incision with 2 malleable retractors placed beneath it. Care should be taken to avoid paratenon stripping, as this is an important structure vital to the nutrition acquisition of the tendon.

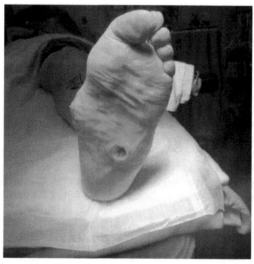

Fig. 6. (Fig.6) This is a preoperative photograph of a 54-year-old man with Charcot Midfoot and unstable, ulcerated, swollen Charcot foot. Note the medial dislocation of cuneiform secondary to Homolateral metatarsal dislocation.

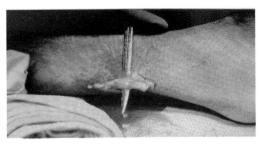

Fig. 7. Open Achilles tendon release. Incision is made midline to the Achilles. A Z-lengthening is performed in the Achilles and free ends are repaired with the surgeon's choice of suture.

The tendon is lengthened using an 11 blade in an anterior to posterior fashion and repaired with a large gauge nonabsorbable suture in a position of neutrality (90° foot to lower leg) as observed on the lateral side of the foot. In some instances, the posterior ankle capsule is also contracted and blocks the correct repositioning of the talus in the mortis. This should be looked for radiographically and addressed with open capsulotomy. The subcutaneous tissue and the skin are both repaired with suture.

Percutaneous lengthening of the Achilles tendon requires careful prone positioning of the patient with the leg properly stabilized, or a strong assistant who can hold the leg aloft for the entirety of the procedure. In this technique, the surgeon can begin by finding the bisection of the Achilles tendon through manual palpation. Once found, a stab incision is made parallel to the long axis of the tendon at least 3 finger widths above the insertion. The foot is pushed in dorsiflexion to apply tension to the tendon. The incision is carried deep through the fibers of the tendon and the blade is turned medially, thus incising half of the tendon from the midline. The second stab incision is likewise made mid-substance, again, 3 finger widths superior to the former. This time, the surgical cut is through and through in the opposite direction, laterally. This produces a "Z" cut allowing for lengthening. The procedure can be repeated up to the myotendinous junction. This alternative percutaneous method is an acceptable alternative to the preferred open tendo-Achilles lengthening.

HINDFOOT PINNING

Once the TAL is complete it is strongly recommended that the hindfoot be stabilized to the tibia for proper further reconstruction of the midfoot to ensue. This is performed using fluoroscopy and proceeds by introducing a Steinmann pin into the plantar tuber of the calcaneus at an acute angle and advancing it until it crosses the posterior tibia and buries itself into the posterior aspect of the tibia. The placement should be checked with fluoroscopy to ensure that the ankle is at neutrality (90°) and the calcaneus demonstrates a positive inclination angle (**Fig. 8**).

MIDFOOT OSTEOTOMY

Surgical correction of the Charcot midfoot can now proceed. In this case, an extensile incision is made two fingerbreadths inferior and distal to the medial malleolus and is extended to the mid-shaft of the first metatarsal. The incision is developed thru the subcutaneous tissue dissection and the medial venous structures are carefully protected or ligated as needed. Unless the first metatarsal cuneiform joint is involved in

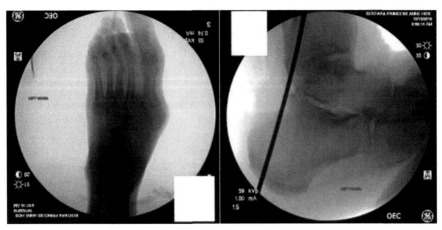

Fig. 8. Open lengthening of the Achilles is favored to achieve adequate length. It is necessary to fix the tendon such that there is a neutral, or 90-degree, relationship between the hindfoot and the leg. Note that the hindfoot is temporarily fixated to the tibia with an extra-articular Steinmann pin. Reconstruction of the Charcot foot begins with this stable hindfoot.

the Charcot destruction, the tibialis anterior can be gently retracted and worked around. In other instances, however, it should be cleanly divided and tagged for reapproximation with nonabsorbable suture during wound closure.

When correcting a Charcot midfoot, the authors' have found that in many instances, a bone has become completely dislocated, as is the case with the medial cuneiform in this example. In such instances, removal of the dislocated bone should be performed. It can then be wrapped in a saline sponge for later reimplantation as occurred here, or placed in a bone mill for additional grafting (**Fig. 9**). In either case, removal of the articular cartilage is recommended.

In this case, the Lisfranc joint is involved in the collapse, as such the bases of the metatarsals and attendant cuneiforms should be prepared for fusion. Arthrodesis of

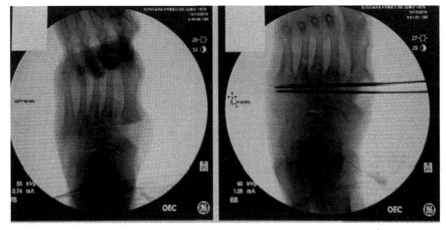

Fig. 9. Medial cuneiform temporarily extirpated, permitting corrective closing wedge osteotomy.

the Lisfranc joint can be accomplished by placing 2 intersecting k-wires across the foot from medial to lateral. The area between the 2 k-wires can be resected using a sagittal saw or sharp osteotome. An envelope containing nerves, blood vessels, tendons, and subcutaneous tissue can be raised off the bone and maintained with army-navy retractors during resection. Fluoroscopy is invaluable during this portion of the repair. This wedge of diseased bone resection provides a raw bone surface optimal for arthrodesis. The talonavicular joint and the subtalar joint can now be prepared for arthrodesis using curettes and sharp osteotomes.

An additional incision is now required on the lateral aspect of the foot over lying the calcaneal cuboid joint. This incision is needed to fully reduce the cuboid, whose plantar dislocation is a constant finding with Charcot foot collapse. That dislocation is at both the calcaneocuboid joint and the cuboid metatarsal articulation. Both must be addressed and anatomically repaired.

The concept of derotation of the mal-aligned midfoot against a stable hindfoot block cannot be over-emphasized (**Fig. 10**). Reconstruction now enters a fixation phase with the placement of a guide pin for the medial column. The guide pin is best placed percutaneously with fluoroscopic assistance into the plantar aspect of the first metatarsal head (**Fig. 11**). If the wire is truly in the medullary canal, it can be advanced without the drill turning by simply pushing it forward. In this case, it was first advanced without replacing the medial cuneiform, creating a linear relationship with the navicular and into the talus. After this was accomplished, the prepared cuneiform was reintroduced into the column and the pin retracted, then again advanced through the same path into the talus.

A key step in anatomic reconstruction is to correct the deformity on the frontal plane while placing the guide pins. The collapse of the medial column can be visualized as the elevation of the first ray segment and the reciprocal plantar position of the lateral column. The medial column requires alignment to recreate the Meary's angle;

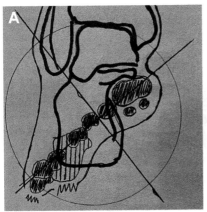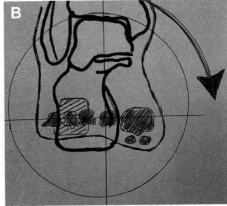

Fig. 10. (*A*) This drawing depicts the resultant position of the midfoot/forefoot subsequent to Charcot foot fracture dislocation. Fracture and ligament failure create a scenario of instability whereby the medial, weight bearing, column fails, elevating up. It's seen as a disruption of Meary's angle. Laterally the midfoot fails with the metatarsal bases dislocating on top of the cuboid pushing it beneath them and creating the classic cuboid ulcer. Please note the drawing depicts an additional ulcer created by the base of the 5th metatarsal. This can be treated with both ostectomy and derotation. (*B*) When derotation is completed, the midfoot is anatomically realigned. This greatly lessens the likelihood of plantar lateral ulceration.

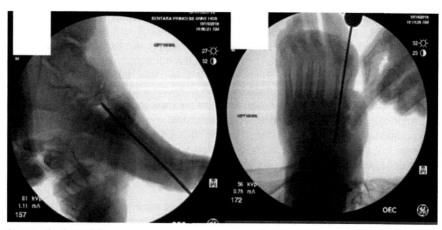

Fig. 11. The lateral fluoroscopy shows stacking now absent; Steinmann pins are placed for cannulated drilling and placement of cannulated beams.

however, the lateral column requires the rotation of the osteotomy to elevate the lateral column. Otherwise, the lateral column may be left in a position with the cuboid and styloid process of the 5th metatarsal inferior to their correct alignment; recurrent ulceration is a potential result. With this step completed, a lateral column guide pin for a beam can be placed under fluoroscopy. It is the authors' preference to place the lateral beam parallel to the supporting surface and introduce the guide pin between the bases of the flared 3rd and 4th metatarsals. This position fuses both the Lisfranc joint and the calcaneocuboid joint (**Fig. 12**A and **Fig. 12**B).

Application of Hardware

The Charcot foot correction now progresses with the addition of 2 necessary beams. Application of medial and lateral beams prohibits the recurrence of deformity. A sagittal plane fluoroscopic image will reveal any remaining deformity such as stacking

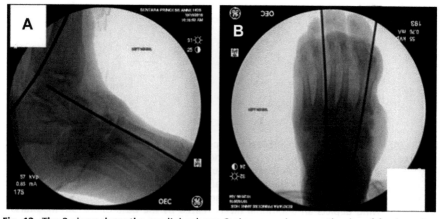

Fig. 12. The 2 views show the medial column Steinmann pin correctly placed for beaming. The lateral column can now be rotated around it into an anatomic alignment and percutaneously pinned. The AP view shows ideal placement of the 2 Steinmann pins.

of the metatarsals. With the alignment in a satisfactory position, the hardware can be applied (**Figs. 13** and **14**).

APPLICATION OF SUPPLEMENTAL BEAMS

Additional fixation is recommended for Charcot foot reconstruction and is evidenced in the literature through better postoperative outcomes.[14,15] As the underlying reason for the surgery is a global deficiency in the foot's ligamentous and bone integrity, the possibility of further failure and nonunion or pseudoarthrosis (46% reported in the peer-review literature) is extremely high, the following recommendations can be made[27]:

1. Fusion of the subtalar joint is recommended.
2. The addition of a beaming "Truss" crossing obliquely from the base of one of the medial column metatarsals into the body of the calcaneus creates a functional triangle within the foot.

Additional fixation is recommended for Charcot foot reconstruction and has been supported in the literature.[14,15,33] Specifically, the subtalar joint should be arthrodesed for 2 reasons. Firstly, we believe the subtalar fusion limits the independent motion of both columns of the foot, and results in loads in one column being shared by the second. This limits motion and migration of hardware and further joint ligament excess motion, which can lead to collapse. Second, the subtalar joint actually can open and fail with increasing loads as referenced in our below listed preliminary study. This is seen as the development of the negative calcaneal inclination angle often seen in collapsed Charcot. Arthrodesis of the subtalar joint should include a large diameter beam placed through the posterior facet and into the talus.

More recently, our team has been augmenting our Charcot reconstructions with an additional novel truss beam, with favorable results. Our anecdotal 3-year postop results identify no migration of hardware or reoccurrence of deformity. We suggest an additional truss beam should be placed between the medial columns of the forefoot (2nd metatarsal base), into the calcaneus. We believe that the oblique placement of this beam causes it to act mechanically as a truss tie rod, holding together and

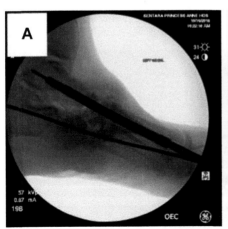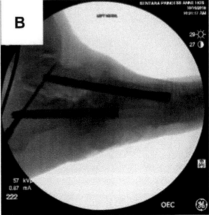

Fig. 13. A sagittal plane fluoroscopic image will reveal any remaining deformity such as stacking of the metatarsals. With the alignment in a satisfactory position, the hardware can be applied.

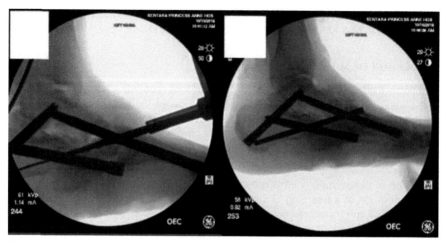

Fig. 14. The placement of the subtalar beam for Arthrodesis inhibits subtalar dislocation. The beam across the columns from medial to lateral creates a truss or tie rod, holding the anatomic relationship between the medial column beam and the subtalar beam.

maintaining the relationship of the medial column beam to the subtalar beam. In doing so, it maintains the positive calcaneal inclination angle and a zero degree Meary's angles. In engineering, we define a truss as a structural member usually fabricated from a straight piece of metal or timber to form a triangle lying in a single plane. Triangle trusses are the simplest and are used to evenly distribute the weight among 2 adjacent beams (**Fig. 15**). The triangle is the strongest shape in physics and of all triangles, the strongest is an equilateral. Unfortunately, the creation of equilateral triangulation may be difficult to accomplish due to the regional anatomy; however, almost as strong is the isosceles triangle with 2 equal-length sides. The isosceles shape should be the goal when placing the beam acting as a truss. The addition of a truss provides a vital but simple added point of fixation to make the construct much stronger and resist failure. It can be placed via open or percutaneous methods.

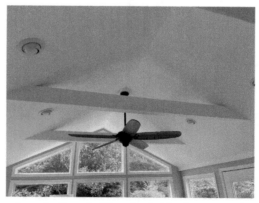

Fig. 15. A tie rod portion of a Truss holding the 2 sides from spreading out, and directing the force to the load-bearing walls.

Preliminary Validation of Truss Model

The possibility of testing different Charcot constructs via a simple model was investigated on a preliminary basis. The experiment methods used an anatomic articulated PVC foot model. This early anatomic study focused on maximum force causing deflection. This model was theorized to mimic the Charcot foot with incompetent ligaments. The model was affixed firmly to a test jig made from an Ilizarov three-ring external fixator and free weights.

The talar body was potted into the custom jig and secured into place to the top ring. The foot was potted into place on Plastazote to increase the friction of the model-ground interface. The center ring was then attached to the top ring by sliding connecting rods that could be variously held tight or completely released. The foot model was "beamed" with various placements of small diameter Kirschner wires placed with a k-driver under fluoroscopy.

The following constructs of k-wire placement were selected (**Fig. 16**):

A. Medial Column only (First Metatarsal head to Talus)
B. Medial Column + Calcaneal-Cuboid Arthrodesis
C. Charcot Triple (Medial Column + Calcaneal-Cuboid Arthrodesis + STJ)
D. Charcot Triple + Truss (2nd metatarsal base to the body of the Calcaneus)

Using a mini c-arm for radiographic observation, the test jig was applied to one of the four above-described models (**Fig. 17**). Using the "live run time" feature of the mini c-arm, 2.5lb weights were incrementally applied to the test models. Imaging was recorded using the sagittal view in an analysis of failure. Failure was defined as the wire bending or yielding under the defined increment of weight. All models were tested and retested for frame inter-rated reliability. Once force testing was performed on all models, x-rays were printed and angular and positional changes were quantified with goniometers as seen in the below radiographs (**Fig. 18**).

In test subject "A," preload radiographs demonstrated congruity of all joints without medial Kirschner wire failure (**Fig. 19**A). The model was then subjected to 2.5lb of weight, which resulted in faulting at both unfixated joints (CC and STJ) (**Fig. 19**B). From this analysis, we identify that the bending moment is resisted at the TN joint

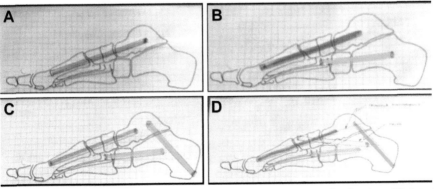

Fig. 16. (*A*) A test model with only a medial column Kirschner wire for fixation. (*B*) A test model with medial and lateral column Kirschner wire for fixation. (*C*) A test model with medial and lateral column Kirschner wire with the addition of a subtalar Kirschner wire for fixation. (*D*) A test model with medial, lateral, subtalar, and "truss" Kirschner wire for fixation.

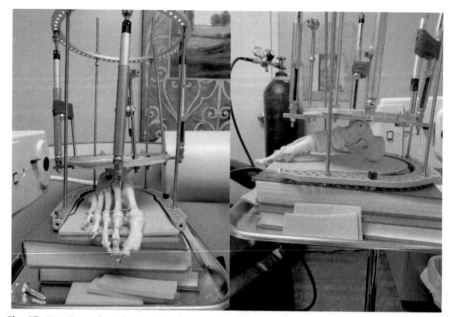

Fig. 17. Test jig as described. A platform can accommodate weights from free weight set in 2.5 lb. increments. Mini c arm can be positioned to obtain fluoroscopic images of articulated PVC model "beamed" with simple Kirschner wires.

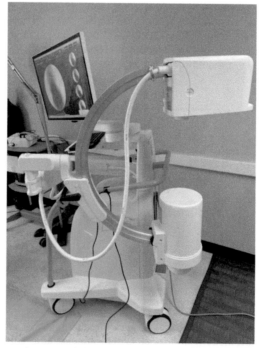

Fig. 18. Mini c-arm used to record data.

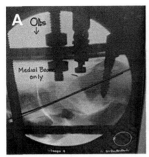
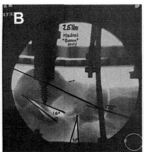
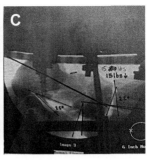

Fig. 19. Test subject "A" with medial column Kirschner wire only. Image (A) demonstrates preload imaging, before the addition of weight. Image (B) depicts the application of 2.5lb of weight. Note the faulting of the CC joint and subtalar joint. Image (C) Identified the weight (15lb) related to the material deformation of the medial column Kirschner wire and the failure of the construct.

but is "seen" in all other unfixated areas. The model has exposed to incremental additions of 2.5lb until such a time that the medial Kirschner wire demonstrated faulting or failure (**Fig. 19**C). The medial wire reached mechanical failure at 15lb. This failure represents the weight that the material and diameter are able to resist before deformation.

In test subject "B," a Kirschner wire placed along the medial and lateral column was tested in a similar fashion (**Fig. 20**). A preload image was taken to ensure congruity of the joints before the application of load. The model was then incrementally loaded until faulting of hardware was noted via radiographs. As predicted, the model with the addition of a second beam, resisted deformation at a higher load, suggesting that the supplementary beams increase the stability of the surgical construct.

In test subject "C," Kirschner wires were applied along both the medial and lateral column as well as the subtalar joint and were tested in a similar fashion as described above. Preload radiographs indicate congruity of all joints without mechanical faulting (**Fig. 21**A). Incremental application of 2.5lbs was performed until mechanical failure of

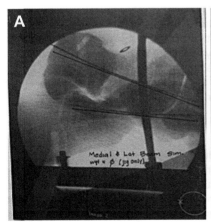
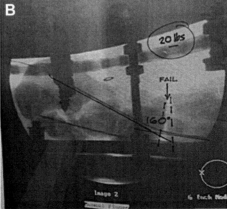

Fig. 20. Test subject "B" with medial column Kirschner wire and lateral column Kirschner wire. Image (A) demonstrates preload imaging before the addition of weight. Image (B) Identified the weight (20lb) related to the material deformation of the medial column Kirschner wire and the failure of the construct.

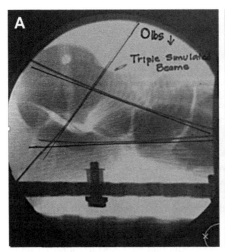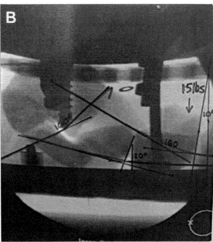

Fig. 21. Test subject "C" with medial and lateral columns well as subtalar Kirschner wires. Image (*A*) demonstrates preload imaging before the addition of weight. Image (*B*) identified the weight (15lb) related to the material deformation of all the Kirschner wires and faulting of the subtalar, calcaneal-cuboid, and naviculocuneiform joint.

wire was identified via x-ray (**Fig. 21**B). Interestingly, mechanical failure of subject "C" was at a lower load (15 lbs.) than test subject "B" and demonstrated failure at all 3 Kirschner wires and their attendant joints. This suggests that the weight is shared evenly throughout the foot and that likely the subtalar joint acts to unite the medial and lateral columns.

In test subject "D," Kirschner wires were applied along medial, lateral columns, subtalar joint, and from the base of the 2nd metatarsal into the calcaneal body (truss). A preload image was taken to ensure congruity of all joints (**Fig. 22**A). The model was then incrementally loaded until faulting of the hardware was noted via radiographic evidence (**Fig. 22**B). As predicted, the truss model with the addition of the fourth beam, resisted deformation at the highest weights.

This preliminary study identifies some obvious features of Charcot repair. The more beams used will add rigidity to the construct and resist deformation and mechanical failure. What remains unclear from this study is the actual changes in loads that can be expected when the test material is changed from Kirschner wires to actual Charcot grade implants. Further research is required to identify the best structural configuration to resist hardware failure and reoccurrence of deformity.

WHEN BEAMS FAIL

Currently, the literature does reveal beam failure with Charcot repair, and the need for revision surgery. The reasons are multi factorial but include: material weakness of the beam, insufficient sizing of the beam, and insufficient screw configuration. With regard to the material strength of hardware, titanium has many applications in foot and ankle surgery. However, it is not nearly as strong as stainless steel in yield strength. Furthermore, the tensile strength of titanium at failure is 31,900 psi; compared with stainless steel valued at 450,000 psi. Shear stress is another measure of a material whereby comparisons can be drawn. Titanium shear stress is rated 240 to 335 MPa; stainless steel, however, is rated at 74.5 to 597 MPa, making stainless steel more likely to resist

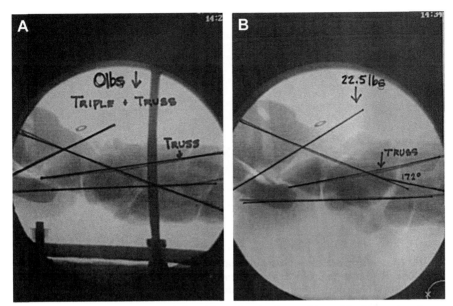

Fig. 22. Test subject "C" with medial and lateral, subtalar, and truss Kirschner wires. Image (*A*) demonstrates preload imaging before the addition of weight. Image (*B*) identified the weight (22.5lb) related to the material deformation of the medial Kirschner wire and faulting of the naviculocuneiform joint. Note there is no change in the position of the foot.

this force. Charcot-specific implants should clearly be made from surgical stainless screws, as they are materially stronger to resist the loads seen in the Charcot midfoot.

Many standard orthopedic screws, that have in the past been used to beam, have core diameters insufficient for protection against non–union-related failures. A traditional screw has a known geometric pattern, which aids in the compression of bone. The features of a traditional screw have a robust thread pattern followed by a much smaller core diameter, which helps to support interfragmentary compression. A traditional beam is not made as a tapered device and works best with a known geometric diameter. For example, an 8.0 mm threaded screw may have an 8.0 mm thread diameter but has a core diameter of only 4.0 - 4.5 mm. This core diameter is likely insufficient to support the mechanical needs of a collapsing Charcot midfoot, as was described earlier in our discussion of bending moment force. An additional engineering concept used in the creation of an appropriately sized beam is the calculation of a section modulus. Section modulus is a geometric property for the cross-sectional design of beams. It is a ratio of the maximum moment on a beam and the maximum fiber stress. It is used to find the minimum required beam diameter that will support a given bending load. This calculation for a circular beam is as follows (**Fig. 23**): whereby

$$Z = \left(\frac{\pi}{4R}\right)(R^4 - R_i^4).$$

Fig. 23. The equation for section modulus of a rod. This equation aids in the identification of the cross-sectional geometric requirements of a beam.

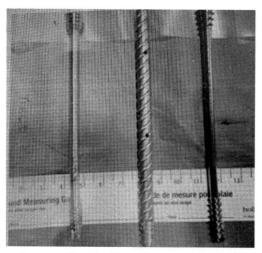

Fig. 24. The 2 orthopedic screws (flanking) have been removed from a failed Charcot reconstructions after undergoing yield, and deforming. Note that their section modulus is much smaller than a Charcot-specific implant (center).

"Z" is section modulus and "R" is the radius. Clearly, a larger section modulus means a stronger beam with all other factors being equal. The following photograph of 2 orthopedic screws used as beams compared with a Charcot-specific prototype design shows a clear difference in section modulus (**Fig. 24**). Notice that both screws, from different manufacturers, went on to yield, (see the fixed bowing along their shafts). Yield is what happens to a beam before complete failure, and is defined as the load at which a solid material begins to change shape permanently. Notice both orthopedic screws went to yield because their core diameters and section modulus are much smaller than the Charcot-specific prototype beam. When we look at human anatomy, we see similar design architecture in the foot. **Fig. 25** shows that at joints whereby the bending moments are greatest. The slender metatarsal flares at its base, markedly increasing its section modulus. Similarly, the navicular also flares whereby it articulates with the talus. These joints were designed to respect these engineering principles.

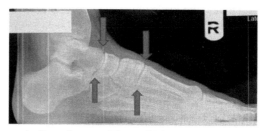

Fig. 25. The red arrows indicated areas of flare which evidence natural occurring alterations in the section modulus. This increase in width aids in support of the medial column.

SUMMARY

Beaming the Charcot foot has its origins and its future in the hands of determined podiatric surgeons. It is a solution to a metabolic bone disease, based on the fundamental principles of podiatric biomechanics, engineering science, material science, and 19th-century railroad trestle design. It respects the soft tissue envelope, and indeed is a superconstruct, without necessarily requiring extensive dissection. As percutaneous corrections of the deformity progress, beaming is the likely solution for most Charcot reconstructions. Similar to endovascular procedures for diabetic peripheral vascular disease, the accomplished diabetic foot, and ankle surgeon will need to master beaming to offer their most compromised patients the chance for limb salvage and continued bipedal gait.

DISCLOSURE

William Grant Medical Consultant for OrthofixLisa Grant-McDonald Medical Consultant for Orthofix.

REFERENCES

1. Svendsen OL, Rabe OC, Winther-Jensen M, et al. How common is the rare charcot foot in patients with diabetes? Diabetes Care 2021;44(4):e62–3.
2. Gilchrist JA, Best CH, Banting FG. Observations with insulin on department of soldiers' civil Re-establishment diabetics. Can Med Assoc J 1923;13(8): 565–72.
3. Banting FG, Campbell WR, Fletcher AA. Further clinical experience with insulin (pancreatic extracts) in the treatment of diabetes mellitus. Br Med J 1923; 1(3236):8–12.
4. Orioli L, Hammer F, Vande Berg B, et al. Prevalence, characteristics, and prognosis of peripheral arterial disease in patients with diabetic charcot foot. J Foot Ankle Surg 2021;60(6):1158–63.
5. Pakarinen TK, Laine HJ, Maenpaa H, et al. Long-term outcome and quality of life in patients with Charcot foot. Foot Ankle Surg 2009;15(4):187–91.
6. Pinzur MS, Evans A. Health-related quality of life in patients with Charcot foot. Am J Orthop (Belle Mead Nj) 2003;32(10):492–6.
7. Raspovic KM, Hobizal KB, Rosario BL, et al. Midfoot charcot neuroarthropathy in patients with diabetes: the impact of foot ulceration on self-reported quality of life. Foot Ankle Spec 2015;8(4):255–9.
8. Sochocki MP, Verity S, Atherton PJ, et al. Health related quality of life in patients with Charcot arthropathy of the foot and ankle. Foot Ankle Surg 2008; 14(1):11–5.
9. Albright RH, Joseph RM, Wukich DK, et al. Is reconstruction of unstable midfoot charcot neuroarthropathy cost effective from a US payer's perspective? Clin Orthop Relat Res 2020;478(12):2869–88.
10. Zhou HB, Zhang C, Liu CL, et al. [Clinical observation on plate on the metatarsal side to reconstruction of tarsometatarsal joint dislocations secondary to diabetic charcot foot]. Zhongguo Gu Shang 2016;29(6):553–6.
11. Ramadani F, Haragus H, Radu P, et al. [Complex reconstruction with internal locking plate fixation for Charcot arthropathy]. Orthopade 2015;44(1):33–8.
12. Garchar D, DiDomenico LA, Klaue K. Reconstruction of Lisfranc joint dislocations secondary to Charcot neuroarthropathy using a plantar plate. J Foot Ankle Surg 2013;52(3):295–7.

13. Sammarco VJ. Superconstructs in the treatment of charcot foot deformity: plantar plating, locked plating, and axial screw fixation. Foot Ankle Clin 2009;14(3): 393–407.

14. Grant WP, Garcia-Lavin S, Sabo R. Beaming the columns for Charcot diabetic foot reconstruction: a retrospective analysis. J Foot Ankle Surg 2011;50(2): 182–9.

15. Grant WP, Garcia-Lavin SE, Sabo RT, et al. A retrospective analysis of 50 consecutive Charcot diabetic salvage reconstructions. J Foot Ankle Surg 2009; 48(1):30–8.

16. Folestad A, Alund M, Asteberg S, et al. Role of Wnt/beta-catenin and RANKL/OPG in bone healing of diabetic Charcot arthropathy patients. Acta Orthop 2015;86(4):415–25.

17. La Fontaine J, Harkless LB, Sylvia VL, et al. Levels of endothelial nitric oxide synthase and calcitonin gene-related peptide in the Charcot foot: a pilot study. J Foot Ankle Surg 2008;47(5):424–9.

18. Mabilleau G, Petrova N, Edmonds ME, et al. Number of circulating CD14-positive cells and the serum levels of TNF-alpha are raised in acute charcot foot. Diabetes Care 2011;34(3):e33.

19. Ndip A, Williams A, Jude EB, et al. The RANKL/RANK/OPG signaling pathway mediates medial arterial calcification in diabetic Charcot neuroarthropathy. Diabetes 2011;60(8):2187–96.

20. Witzke KA, Vinik AI, Grant LM, et al. Loss of RAGE defense: a cause of Charcot neuroarthropathy? Diabetes Care 2011;34(7):1617–21.

21. La Fontaine J, Shibuya N, Sampson HW, et al. Trabecular quality and cellular characteristics of normal, diabetic, and charcot bone. J Foot Ankle Surg 2011; 50(6):648–53.

22. Wiewiorski M, Yasui T, Miska M, et al. Solid bolt fixation of the medial column in Charcot midfoot arthropathy. J Foot Ankle Surg 2013;52(1):88–94.

23. Butt DA, Hester T, Bilal A, et al. The medial column Synthes Midfoot Fusion Bolt is associated with unacceptable rates of failure in corrective fusion for Charcot deformity: results from a consecutive case series. Bone Joint J 2015;97-B(6): 809–13.

24. Lowery NJ, Woods JB, Armstrong DG, et al. Surgical management of Charcot neuroarthropathy of the foot and ankle: a systematic review. Foot Ankle Int 2012;33(2):113–21.

25. Shazadeh Safavi P, Jupiter DC, Panchbhavi V. A systematic review of current surgical interventions for charcot neuroarthropathy of the midfoot. J Foot Ankle Surg 2017;56(6):1249–52.

26. Schneekloth BJ, Lowery NJ, Wukich DK. Charcot neuroarthropathy in patients with diabetes: an updated systematic review of surgical management. J Foot Ankle Surg 2016;55(3):586–90.

27. Ford SE, Cohen BE, Davis WH, et al. Clinical outcomes and complications of midfoot charcot reconstruction with intramedullary beaming. Foot Ankle Int 2019; 40(1):18–23.

28. Cates NK, Furmanek J, Dubois KS, et al. Risk factors and outcomes after surgical reconstruction of charcot neuroarthropathy in fracture versus dislocation patterns. J Foot Ankle Surg 2021;61(2):264–71.

29. Richter M, Mittlmeier T, Rammelt S, et al. Intramedullary fixation in severe Charcot osteo-neuroarthropathy with foot deformity results in adequate correction without loss of correction - results from a multi-centre study. Foot Ankle Surg 2015;21(4): 269–76.

30. Wukich DK, Liu GT, Raspovic K, et al. Biomechanical performance of charcot-specific implants. J Foot Ankle Surg 2021;60(3):440–7.
31. Grant WP, Sullivan R, Sonenshine DE, et al. Electron microscopic investigation of the effects of diabetes mellitus on the Achilles tendon. J Foot Ankle Surg 1997; 36(4):272–8 [discussion: 330].
32. Colen LB, Kim CJ, Grant WP, et al. Achilles tendon lengthening: friend or foe in the diabetic foot? Plast Reconstr Surg 2013;131(1):37e–43e.
33. Manchanda K, Wallace SB, Ahn J, et al. Charcot midfoot reconstruction: does subtalar arthrodesis or medial column fixation improve outcomes? J Foot Ankle Surg 2020;59(6):1219–23.

The Use of Hexapod External Fixation in the Management of Charcot Foot and Ankle Deformities

Guido A. LaPorta, DPM, MS, FACFAS[a],*, Maria Begum, DPM[b],
Stephanie Guzelak, DPM[b], Alison D'Andelet, DPM, MHA[c]

KEYWORDS

- Charcot foot and ankle deformities • External fixation • Intramedullary beaming
- Mitter frame • Butt frame • Computer hexapod–assisted podiatric surgery

KEY POINTS

- Benefits of circular external fixation are the ability to provide triplane stability while addressing deformities that may be occurring in multiple planes or at multiple levels.
- Accuracy of correction is enhanced by the ability to perform postcorrection "residuals".
- Computer hexapod–assisted podiatric surgery (CHAPS) additionally allows deformity correction while minimizing surgical dissection and bone resection and therefore potentially minimizing the need for bone grafts.
- External fixation can be used in conjunction with internal fixation (neutralization frame) to enhance stability or in presence of osteomyelitis in the midfoot secondary to ulceration.
- 10 Hexapod rules are vital to proper multiplanar deformity.

INTRODUCTION

Charcot neuroarthropathy (CN) is a devastating and disabling pathology in the foot and ankle, which predominately affects the midfoot, in well-recognized patterns, and also the ankle and hindfoot joints. Of the 30.3 million people in the United States currently diagnosed with diabetes, approximately 0.5% (0.08%–7.5%) will develop CN at some point in their lives.[1,2] This results in loss of normal pedal architecture, gait dysfunction, and soft tissue compromise. Sanders and Frykberg, as well as

a Podiatric Medical Education, Our Lady of Lourdes Memorial Hospital, Binghamton, NY 13905, USA; b Podiatric Medical Education, Our Lady of Lourdes Memorial Hospital, Attention: Graduate Medical Education, 169 Riverside Drive, Binghamton, NY 13905, USA; c Upper Chesapeake Medical Center, Bel Air, MD 21014, USA
* Corresponding author. 414 East Drinker Street, Dunmore, PA 18512, USA
E-mail address: Glaporta@msn.com

Clin Podiatr Med Surg 39 (2022) 629–642
https://doi.org/10.1016/j.cpm.2022.05.010
0891-8422/22/© 2022 Elsevier Inc. All rights reserved.
podiatric.theclinics.com

Brodsky, classified the anatomic patterns of involvement in CN, and determined that the tarsometatarsal joints and/or midtarsal joints are most commonly involved.[3,4] The prevalence of the deformity at this anatomic location prompted Schon and Sammarco to each further classify midfoot Charcot in 1998.[5] Progressive subluxation and dislocation of the midfoot frequently leads to the development of a "rocker-bottom" deformity. Progressive subluxation and dislocation of the lateral column is the hallmark of end-stage midfoot CN and is very difficult to correct and maintain correction. The Schon Classification describes additional features, which are useful in planning treatment strategies. The midfoot types all start medially and progress laterally. Type I starts at the first, second, and third metatarsal cuneiform joints producing a plantar prominence resulting in an early, medial ulcer. The predominant forefoot position is abduction. Type II starts at the navicular cuneiform joint, higher in the vault of the arch, and therefore the plantar prominence is more central and lateral. The ulcer begins more lateral and may progress from central to medial. The predominant position of the forefoot is abducted. Types I and II look similar clinically but the delayed ulcer formation in type II, which does not occur until there is lateral column instability, may delay aggressive intervention. Type I intervention occurs early in the disease process because the ulcer forms early. Type III is perinavicular and predominantly involves the navicular cuneiform and talonavicular joints due to collapse and fragmentation of the navicular. The predominant position of the foot is forefoot adduction, which results in central to lateral plantar ulcer formation. Type IV involves the transverse tarsal joint, predominately the talonavicular joint, which results in a more medial or central ulcer. The predominant position of the foot is forefoot abduction with excessive weight-bearing medially on the talar head. Frequently, ulcers form on the plantar medial aspect of the talar head. Infection of the underlying talus may be the nexus for extension of the disease process to the ankle. In addition, the presence of an equinus contracture deformity secondary to motor and sensory neuropathy and subsequent motor imbalance can increase forces through the midfoot, further contributing to collapse.[6] The Achilles tendon in diabetic patients is subject to glycation of collagen fibers, which leads to increased stiffness and higher peak plantar pressures.[7] Abnormal plantar pedal pressure and shearing forces increase the risk of ulceration, osteomyelitis, and possible amputation.[8] A study by Sohn and colleagues found that diabetic patients with CN alone had a risk of amputation 7 times greater than patients with neuropathic foot ulcerations, and a risk of amputation 12 times greater if they had an ulcer secondary to the Charcot deformity.[9] Thus, patients with midfoot CN, particularly those with current or prior ulceration, are at high risk for infection, amputation, and even mortality if the deformity is not addressed.

Ankle joint CN presents unique problems involving instability and deformity, which have proven difficult to treat with bracing. The disease may affect the tibial articular surface resulting in varus instability and lateral ulceration. In addition, the talus may present with avascular necrosis or osteomyelitis leading to valgus instability and medial ulceration. Frequently, there is complete dissolution of the talus, which requires excision of the remaining bone and fusion of the tibial-calcaneal interface. These presentations are complicated by ankle joint contracture and equinus deformity. Longstanding deformity frequently leads to subtalar joint involvement if not frank dislocation. This ankle-hindfoot instability is accompanied by ulceration, lower extremity edema, and soft tissue or bone infection. These variables render the extremity difficult to brace, which frequently results in patients becoming sedentary and unable or unwilling to participate in activities of daily living. The authors consider patients with ankle CN to present a primary surgical problem.

INDICATIONS FOR USE OF HEXAPOD FIXATION

The use of circular external fixation follows an orderly thought process. If the deformity can be completely corrected acutely, static external fixation can be used as either the primary fixation or as a compliment to internal fixation (neutralization frame). If residual deformity persists following acute correction, a dynamic frame using hinges and motors is useful. A forefoot ring connected to a Butt frame construct with 4 hinged struts ("Steering wheel" technique) is very useful for correction of midfoot Charcot. If the deformity is multilevel or multiplanar, hexapod external fixation is indicated.

The perceived benefits of circular external fixation are the ability to provide triplane stability while addressing deformities that may be occurring in multiple planes or at multiple levels. In addition, there may be segmental bone loss complicated by infection and acquired leg length discrepancies. Joint contractures can be managed as well as control and protection of the soft tissue envelope. Based on the type of external fixation construct, all the above may be done on an acute or gradual basis.

Computer hexapod–assisted podiatric surgery (CHAPS) additionally allows deformity correction while minimizing surgical dissection and bone resection and therefore potentially minimizing the need for bone grafts. Gradual correction may encourage earlier intervention while protecting the soft tissue and maintaining or restoring length. Accuracy of correction is enhanced by the ability to perform postcorrection "residuals." Hexapod construct types are outlined in Table x.[10]

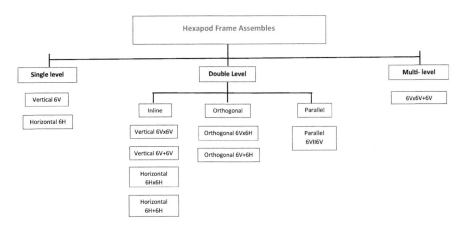

The following hexapod rules are inviolate.

1. Regardless of how complicated a frame looks, the active part consists of 2 rings (partial rings, foot plate) connected by 6 struts.
2. There is always a proximal ring and a distal ring.
3. The software expects that the rings be attached in a certain manner. The master tab (alignment tab, reference tab) is always on the proximal ring and in the case of the tibia, directly opposite the tibial crest.
4. Struts 1 and 2 are always attached to the "master tab" on the proximal ring and proceed around the ring counterclockwise.
5. Either ring (proximal or distal) can be designated the reference ring. The reference ring represents the stationary fragment. The opposite ring represents the moving fragment.

6. With few exceptions, the master tab on foot constructs is rotated 180° to the tibial crest and therefore is located on the plantar aspect of the heel.
7. When viewed from the toes, the struts on the foot construct proceed clockwise.
8. In foot constructs, the distal ring is usually the reference ring.
9. Foot deformities can be planned with and without software.
10. Frame constructs can be either prebuilt or placed on the extremity "rings first."

In addition, each hexapod system has specific rules, regulations, and procedures peculiar to that system. Surgeons should be thoroughly familiar with one system to realize its full potential.

TREATMENT GOALS

The goals in treating CN are to create a stable extremity and plantigrade foot, healing of all neuropathic wounds, and eradication of infection. In addition, the patient should be able to wear a shoe or brace and function as a community ambulator. These goals may be difficult to achieve with conservative treatment in patients with midfoot or ankle pathology because of the propensity of the neuropathic tissue to ulcerate, as well as the difficulty in finding effective and comfortable bracing or shoe gear to accommodate the plantar prominence in rocker-bottom deformity.[11,12] Surgical reconstruction of the foot and ankle for limb salvage is often required to restore function and decrease the risk of amputation secondary to ulceration and infection.

Many procedures have been used in the treatment of midfoot and ankle deformities. Plantar exostectomy, Achilles tendon lengthening, realignment of advanced deformity, ankle and hindfoot arthrodesis, and talectomy with tibial-calcaneal fusion with internal and/or external fixation are all strategies used to address this complex deformity. There is no convincing evidence in the literature that suggests the superiority of any surgical intervention or fixation technique. We present a computer hexapod–assisted 2-stage approach to CN of the foot and ankle which incorporates the basic principles of deformity correction, management of closed or open fracture-dislocations, bone and soft tissue infections, and segmental bone defects. The basic principles of this 2-stage approach have been developed and improved in more than 600 cases with consistent and reproducible results.

SURGICAL TECHNIQUES—MIDFOOT CHARCOT

Midfoot CN pathology can be addressed with either a Butt frame or Miter frame.

Surgical correction of midfoot CN is achieved via the 2-stage technique. The first step of this technique involves acute correction of ankle joint contracture (equinus deformity) and maintenance of that correction during gradual correction of the midfoot deformity using computer hexapod–assisted external fixation. An Achilles tendon lengthening is performed first in order to allow the rearfoot to be placed in a neutral position. Motion at the ankle is monitored on C-arm to ensure that dorsiflexion is occurring at the ankle joint. If adequate correction is achieved at the ankle joint, a Butt frame construct can be used. If the ankle joint is not sufficiently corrected, it may be necessary to use a Miter fame construct. If a Butt frame construct is chosen, the corrected equinus deformity is maintained by placing a 4.0 to 5.0 half pin down the long axis of the calcaneus. This is necessary to achieve anatomic realignment of the midfoot without losing any of the equinus correction. We prefer to perform an open Achilles tendon lengthening. A percutaneous lengthening may be indicated if significant equinus deformity is present, because of the ability to achieve a greater amount of lengthening.[13] Tenotomy, however, runs the risk of producing a calcaneal gait. The

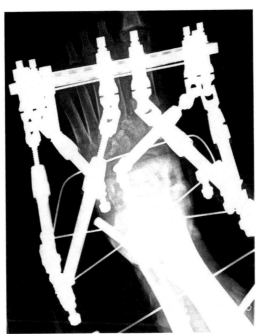

Fig. 1. The construct is applied "Rings First" with the distal ring designated as the Reference Ring and the Master Tab rotated 180° so that it is located on the plantar aspect of the foot.

Achilles tendon lengthening is performed via a midline incision to reduce the risk of complications to the neurovascular structures along the lateral aspect of the gastrocnemius aponeurosis.

The authors prefer gradual correction and realignment because it allows for simultaneous correction of significant multiplanar deformities while maintaining or restoring foot length and bone mass and reducing risk of neurovascular compromise. This approach can be used in *both an* acute or coalesced deformity; however, an osteotomy is required if the deformity is coalesced to allow for anatomic reduction of the bony segments. Ideally, the osteotomy should be placed at the level of the deformity apex to allow for accurate, anatomic correction. In actuality, the osteotomy can only be performed within the confines of the lesser tarsus regardless of whether or not it corresponds with the deformity apex. It is our preference to perform minimally invasive osteotomies in patients with a coalesced deformity. This can be achieved with power saw and osteotome, Gigli saw, and even ultrasound cutting tools. Osteotomies may not be necessary in more acute stages where there is bony dissolution, severe comminution, or nonunion of midfoot fractures, as the foot remains unstable and able to be manipulated.

The hexapod external fixator is then applied to gradually distract (lengthen) and realign the bony segments. The most commonly used construct is a 6×6 Butt frame, which allows for gradual correction of the forefoot on a fixed hindfoot. The decision to use a Butt frame is predicated on the fact that the ankle joint contracture (equinus) has been corrected and the hindfoot osseous architecture is normal or has been acutely corrected. It may be necessary to fuse the subtalar joint to produce a stabile hindfoot. The Butt frame technique used is described as a "rings-first," distal reference, 180-degree offset, 6×6 hexapod (**Fig. 1**). Once the frame components are in place, orthogonal C-arm imaging is used to obtain images of the foot before attaching the 6 hexapod

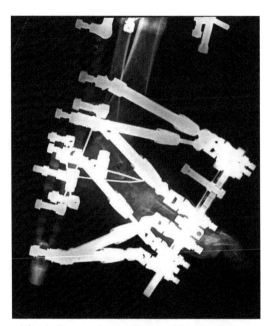

Fig. 2. Correction and final alignment typically take 17 to 24 days.

struts. This imaging provides the deformity parameter information required by the software program to provide a prescription with daily strut adjustments. As the struts are adjusted, the midfoot deformity is realigned over a 17- to 28-day period (**Fig. 2**). Once realignment is achieved, the patient is returned to the operating room for stage 2.

Two additional strategies are used to enhance stability and accuracy. First, vertically tensioned wires can be used to attach the forefoot ring to the metatarsals. This allows multiple wires to be used at relative right angles to each other, which provides a very stable connection of the forefoot ring to the skeleton. Secondly, stirrup wires should be used to enhance deformity correction. Stirrup wires are nontensioned wires placed posterior and anterior to an osteotomy to ensure separation at the desired level. This strategy is important in deformities that present with unstable tarsal joints.

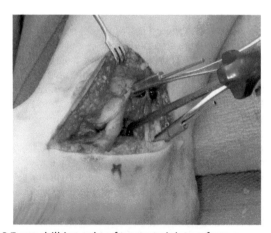

Fig. 3. A flexible 2.7-mm drill is used to fenestrate joint surfaces.

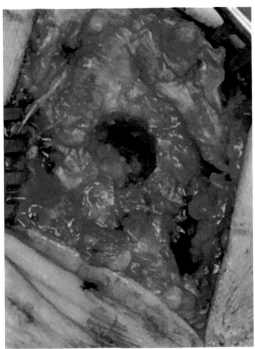

Fig. 4. Joint surfaces may be prepared with trephine and dowel bone graft to facilitate fusion.

The second stage involves removal of the external fixation device, preparation of all joints to be fused, and minimally invasive antegrade or retrograde beaming of the medial and lateral columns. Joint preparation can be achieved by minimally invasive side cutting burrs, or joint resection techniques via multiple short incisions at each joint location. Joint surfaces may be resected via rongeur, sagittal saw, or trephine technique, and a flexible 2.0 to 2.7 mm drill bit is used to fenestrate the subchondral bone (**Fig. 3**). If a trephine technique is used, the subsequent deficit can be packed with bone matrix or autogenous or allograft dowel (**Fig. 4**). Platelet-rich plasma or bone marrow aspirate is also frequently used when preparing the joints for beaming.

Beaming of the medial column is accomplished through a dorsal incision, which also facilitates the reduction of digital hammertoes and contractures. The attachments of the medial and lateral collateral and sesamoid suspensory ligaments are released from the metatarsal head. A guide wire from a 7.0/7.3/8.0 mm cannulated screw set is inserted through the distal aspect of the metatarsal head, just below the midpoint, and is carefully driven into the body of the talus. This wire can also be used as a joystick to ensure appropriate alignment along each segment of the medial column. The ultimate position of the guide wire, confirmed on fluoroscopy, passes through the medullary canal of the first metatarsal and through the head, neck, and body of the talus, without violating the ankle or subtalar joints. A cannulated core diameter drill is used within the metatarsal. The appropriately sized over drill is used to prepare the bone to accept the head of the bone screw, which is inserted and then buried into the metatarsal shaft. If antegrade placement is preferred, the original guidewire is advanced through the body of the talus, exiting the foot just lateral to the Achilles' tendon. The appropriate steps are then performed, and the beaming screw is introduced from posterior to anterior extending no further than the posterior half of the first metatarsal. Solid bone screws may also be used. The screw path holes may be prepared with cannulated instruments before insertion of the solid screws.

Lateral column beaming is performed in a similar fashion. The fourth metatarsal is frequently chosen as it is more in line with the cuboid and calcaneus. A dorsal incision is placed over the fourth metatarsal phalangeal joint and the metatarsal head is released from its soft tissue attachments. Cannulated and core diameter drills are used to prepare the drill hole for the appropriately sized bone screw. Frequently, the diameter of the fourth metatarsal is too small to pass a 7.0/7.3/8.0 mm beam and a 5.0/5.5 mm screw must be used. In addition, the fixation may start at the base of the fifth or fourth metatarsal (**Fig. 5**). Adequate position of each step and final

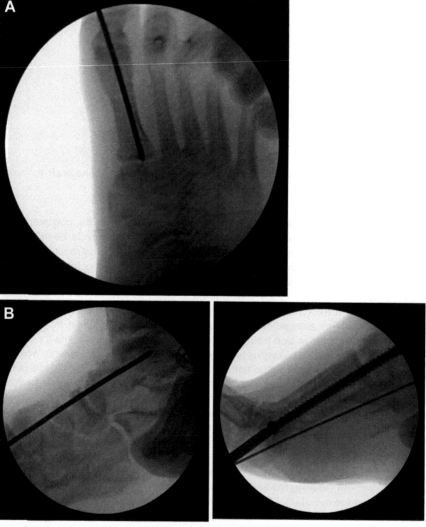

Fig. 5. (*A*) The wire is introduced through the first metatarsal head and directed toward the talar head facilitated by fluoroscopic imaging. (*B*) The wire is placed on a trajectory that allows placement in the talar head and neck.

compression is confirmed with fluoroscopy. Additional intramedullary fixation can be placed as needed through the second or third metatarsal for increased stability. The patient is then placed into a short leg cast with the foot at 90° and may require non–weight-bearing for approximately 10 to 12 weeks. Protected weight-bearing may be allowed based on x-ray appearance on a case-by-case basis.

Alternatively, beaming techniques can be accomplished by specially designed beams or nails specifically designed to withstand the unique shear and bending forces produced by these neuropathic patients.

In cases where the ankle joint contracture is not completely reduced, a Miter frame construct can be used. The Miter frame is a 2-level construct where the miter ring is the distal ring of the tibial construct and the proximal ring of the foot construct. This allows deformity correction at 2 levels, the ankle-hindfoot and also the midfoot. The ankle-hindfoot portion uses a proximal reference ring and is used to correct hindfoot deformity (varus-valgus) and any remaining ankle joint contracture. The foot portion uses a distal reference ring and usually a 180° offset and is used to realign the midfoot deformity. As usual, the miter frame may be retained until final consolidation or removed and replaced with internal fixation.

Alternatively, if the midfoot is not involved, the ankle joint can be addressed with a standard equinus frame that uses a foot plate and tibial ring. This construct can use a proximal or distal reference and in various iterations, is useful for tibial talar, tibial talar calcaneal, or tibial-calcaneal fusions. This construct is loaded in an axial direction and is conducive to early weight-bearing. Alternating compression and distraction maneuvers can be used to improve the fusion mass. Frontal and sagittal plane deformity may be finetuned. In addition, this construct can be used in conjunction with intramedullary nails for enhanced stability.

These techniques can also be modified for cases where osteomyelitis is present in the midfoot secondary to current or prior ulceration. In these cases, all infected bone is resected, and antibiotic beads or spacer are placed in the void during the initial procedure. The antibiotic beads can be absorbable or frequently exchanged before final removal. A hexapod external fixation device can be applied at this time to provide stabilization. Any remaining necrotic soft tissue or bone can also be removed during the first stage. In addition, concern about instability secondary to resection of infected bone is addressed with antibiotic-infused autograft and/or allograft during the second stage of to restore length and provide continued local antibiotic delivery.

DISCUSSION

We approach midfoot and ankle Charcot without ulcer as a closed, noninfected, comminuted, fracture-dislocation with a significant degree of deformity (angulation-translation-rotation) and bony resorption (short significant degree of deformity and bony resorption [shortening]). When an ulcer is present, we approach midfoot and ankle Charcot as an open, infected, comminuted, fracture-dislocation with a significant degree of deformity and bony resorption. We therefore combine the principles of fracture management, musculoskeletal infection, deformity correction, wound healing, and segmental bone defects to manage these most complex deformities.

CN of the midfoot can have a significant effect on patients' ability to function and severely affect the quality of life. There are multiple ways to address midfoot Charcot deformities, but there is no gold standard because of the variety of presentation secondary to acuity, stability, location, and presence of ulceration and/or infection. The various components of the pathology require careful consideration by the surgeon with respect to how best to manage each patient's particular deformity. Regardless of these various components, midfoot Charcot deformity is quite predictable. Regardless of which anatomic type is present, the deformity can be characterized by the following parameters. Sagittal plane abnormality is described as an apex plantar deformity (rocker bottom) and the transverse plane is characterized as an apex medial (ABduction) or apex lateral (ADDuction) deformity. Frontal plane abnormality is typically supinatus regardless of hindfoot position and there is shortening in the axial plane. The goal, however, remains the same regardless of these details—to restore a stable, plantigrade foot, with no ulcerations, which can be placed in a brace or shoe. This 2-stage technique is not presented as a superior method of treating midfoot Charcot, but rather an alternative treatment option that should be considered.

The largest benefit of the 2-stage technique is the complimentary use of internal and external fixation. The use of a hexapod during the first stage provides multiple advantages. The external fixator provides rigid stability to the osseous components and off-loading of the soft tissues, allowing for management of edema and pre-existing soft tissue defects.[14] The computer hexapod–assisted gradual correction achieved during the first stage allows for more accurate anatomic alignment than can be achieved with acute manual reduction, while also providing stability.[15] The hexapod external fixation system has been shown to have a mechanical accuracy within 0.7° and 2 mm and mathematical accuracy of 1/1,000,000 inches in correction of 6-axis deformity.[16] This 2-stage technique is best used in patients who have large angular deformities in multiple planes, or subluxation through the midfoot with or without significant bony defects or fractures, as this technique allows for precise realignment of joints without loss of foot length or bone mass. The gradual correction also protects soft tissue and neurovascular structures often contracted in long-standing deformities and which can be compromised in acute corrections. This allows for minimal incisions and dissection in tissues with poor healing potential.[14,17] The external fixation device also provides the possibility of addressing cases with osteomyelitis, allowing for resection of infected bone, local antibiotic delivery platforms, and subsequent stabilization or deformity correction with placement of internal fixation once the infection is resolved.[14,18]

Significant degree of deformity and bony resorption present inherent challenges in using standard internal fixation techniques to address CN.[19,20] In addition to the poor bone quality, neuropathy, vascular disease, and poor nutrition can delay healing and contribute to complications.[19] These barriers led to the concept of "superconstructs," which are surgical techniques used to improve stability and decrease fixation failure. Superconstructs have 4 defining features: fusion beyond the zone of injury to include normal joints, bony resection to allow for relative shortening of the extremity and adequate deformity reduction without excessive soft tissue tension, use of the strongest possible device tolerated by the soft tissue, and application of the fixation device in a position that maximizes its mechanical function. Axial screw placement, or intramedullary beaming, is one of these superconstructs, along with plantar plating and locking plates.[19] The author prefers to use intramedullary beaming techniques because they have demonstrated noninferiority and can be placed in a percutaneous fashion.

Second stage intramedullary beaming has many advantages compared to plate fixation. Intramedullary beaming allows for the internal fixation device to accept tension on both the dorsal and plantar surfaces, and increases contact area between the bone and fixation, providing increased stability.[20,21] A cadaveric study performed by Pope and colleagues found no significant difference between intramedullary beaming and plantar plating in regards to stiffness, hardware failure, or loads to failure.[22] Thus, the stability benefits of the plantar plate can be achieved with intramedullary beaming without the need for extensive dissection and periosteal stripping that placement of a plantar plate requires.[20,21] The trabecular bone quality present in patients with CN has been found to be weaker and less organized than normal trabecular bone, which can increase failure risk with hardware such as plates or oblique screws due to loss of bone purchase.[23] The intramedullary screw position makes it more inherently stable, even in weaker bone, and also eliminates stress risers in the cortical bone of the metatarsals that can occur with plates or oblique screws.[19] Intramedullary beaming assists in reduction of the deformity, particularly the medial column sag in the sagittal plane, and resists deforming forces within the sagittal and transverse planes[20] restoring Meary's angle. The screws are also placed via small incisions and are completely intraosseous, allowing the bone and soft tissue to act as a biological barrier to protect the hardware in cases of wound dehiscence.[20,24] A study by Cullen and colleagues evaluated use of the midfoot intramedullary nail and experienced an incident in one of their cases in which a deep abscess formed along the lateral incision site, but they were able to maintain the implanted hardware through achievement of bony union because it was not compromised by the soft tissue infection as a plate might have been.[25]

Although intramedullary beaming has proven to be a viable option for the treatment of midfoot Charcot in the literature, there is still some debate regarding the specifics of the screw. The principles of intramedullary nailing in long bones should be applied in this situation in regard to choosing an appropriate size screw. The screw ideally will cross a healthy joint proximal and distal to the affected bones, allowing for a bridging of the area to achieve increased stability. Likewise, the screw should fill the intramedullary canal without compromising the cortical bone, increasing the contact area between the fixation and bone. This generally means that the screw size chosen should be the longest and largest screw able to cross the entire medial or lateral column.[19,21] Typically, this means that screws ranging in size from 6.5 mm to 8.0 mm may not be large enough. Many of the newer beaming systems offer sizes up to 10 mm in diameter.

The material properties of the screws used for midfoot beaming have also been discussed in the literature. It is our preference to use a cannulated system, as it allows for fluoroscopic visualization throughout the placement of the guide wire and screw to ensure appropriate position and alignment. A solid screw, however, must be inserted following removal of a guidewire, which can make placement more technically difficult; however, the path for a solid screw can be prepared using cannulated instrumentation. The benefit of the solid screw is increased strength relative to a cannulated screw. A study by Sammarco and colleagues experienced breakage of 36.4% of their 6.5 mm cannulated screws, whereas studies by Wiewiorski and colleagues and Cullen and colleagues found no breakage of their 6.5 mm solid screws.[25–27] Stainless steel fixation has been shown to have greater tensile strength, greater resistance to load-bearing stress, and longer fatigue failure rate over time when compared to titanium. Titanium has better biocompatibility, improved bone adherence, and absence of allergic response, which may outweigh the limitation of durability in some patients.[20]

The 2-stage technique is also an excellent approach in managing concurrent midfoot CN and osteomyelitis. Osteomyelitis is an additional complicating factor. Abnormal plantar pedal pressure and shearing forces resulting from the midfoot deformity increase the risk of ulceration and osteomyelitis.[8] Patients suspected of having Charcot deformity with osteomyelitis undergo MRI together with bone scintigraphy. An initial leukocyte scan, if positive, is followed by a marrow scan (sulfur colloid). Negative concordance is consistent with osteomyelitis. Positive concordance is consistent with neuroarthropathy without concurrent infection.[28,29] This combined scintigraphy technique improves the diagnostic accuracy in the diabetic foot, with a sensitivity of 92% and specificity of 100%.[28] If osteomyelitis is present, the surgical technique can be modified with the initial stage addressing the infection. The use of a circular external fixation device is indicated during acute or chronic infection and is ideal to stabilize the foot following debridement of infected tissue.[24] Local antibiotic delivery systems are a useful adjunct in these cases as well. The 2 main classes of antibiotic delivery systems are nonbiodegradable systems, such as polymethylmethacrylate (PMMA) beads, and biodegradable systems, such as calcium sulfate/phosphate.[30,31] Although the main disadvantage cited for use of nonbiodegradable systems is the need for additional surgery, it is our preference to use nonbiodegradable systems in these cases as we already plan to return to the operating room for the next stage in the surgical reconstruction. The antibiotics used in these local delivery systems are typically aminoglycosides, which provide good coverage for the most commonly described microbes to cause bone infection, especially chronic osteomyelitis: *Staphylococcus aureus*, Group A beta-hemolytic Streptococcus, Enterobacteriaceae, and *Pseudomonas aeruginosa*.[31] The duration of in vitro elution varies based on the aminoglycoside used, varying from 12 days to 220 days, with the peak elution occurring on the first day.[31]

SUMMARY

The 2-stage computer hexapod–assisted technique is an effective tool to address midfoot Charcot and ankle-hindfoot deformities in order to restore function and decrease the risk of amputation secondary to ulceration and infection. Although this is not the only technique available, it is an excellent option in cases with significant angular deformity or subluxation, need to reduce shortening of the foot, and in the presence of soft tissue defects, with or without concurrent soft tissue or bone infection.

CLINICS CARE POINTS

Pearls:

- The external fixation device also provides the possibility of addressing cases with osteomyelitis, allowing for resection of infected bone, local antibiotic delivery platforms, and subsequent stabilization or deformity correction.

- The osteotomy should be placed at the level of the deformity apex to allow for accurate, anatomic correction. In actuality, the osteotomy can only be performed within the confines of the lesser tarsus regardless of whether or not it corresponds with the deformity apex.

- In addition, each hexapod system has specific rules, regulations, and procedures peculiar to that system. Surgeons should be thoroughly familiar with one system to realize its full potential.

- An Achilles tendon lengthening is performed first to allow the rearfoot to be placed in a neutral position.

- It may be necessary to fuse the subtalar joint to produce a stabile hindfoot.

- When there is potential for delayed healing due to poor bone quality, neuropathy and vascular disease use the concept of "Superconstruct": fusion beyond the zone of injury to include normal joints, bony resection to allow for relative shortening of the extremity and adequate deformity reduction without excessive soft tissue tension, use of the strongest possible device tolerated by the soft tissue, and application of the fixation device in a position that maximizes its mechanical function.

- The screw size should be the longest and largest screw able to cross the entire medial or lateral column for the second stage of the surgery.

Pitfalls:

- Tenotomy to correct equinus deformity can increase the risk of producing a calcaneal gait.
- Position of the guide wire for beam passes through the medullary canal of the first metatarsal and through the head, neck, and body of the talus, without violating the ankle or subtalar joints.
- An osteotomy is required if the deformity is coalesced to allow for anatomic reduction of the bony segments.

DISCLOSURE

The authors have nothing to disclose.

REFERENCES

1. Center for Disease Control/National Center for Chronic Disease Prevention and Health Promotion. National diabetes Statistic Report: Estimates of diabetes and its Burdens in the United States. Atlanta, GA. 2017. Available at: https://www.cdc.gov/diabetes/pdfs/data/statistics/national-diabetes-statistics-report.pdf. Accessed October 5, 2021.
2. Jeffcoate W, Lima J, Nobrega L. The Charcot foot. Diabetic Med 2000;17:253–8.
3. Sanders L, Frykberg RG. Diabetic neuropathic osteoarthropathy: the Charcot foot. The high risk foot in diabetes mellitus. New York: Churchill Livingstone; 1991. p. 297–338.
4. Brodsky JW, Rouse AM. Exostectomy for symptomatic bony prominences in diabetic Charcot feet. Clin Orthop Relat Res 1993;296:21–6.
5. Schon LC, Easley ME, Weinfeld SB. Charcot neuroarthropathy of the foot and ankle. Clinorthop Relat Res 1998;349:116–31.
6. Laborde JM, Philbin TM, Chandler PJ, et al. Preliminary results of primary gastrocnemius-soleus recession for midfoot Charcot arthropathy. Foot and Ankle Specialist 2016;9(2):140–4.
7. Couppe Christian, Svensson Rene Svensson, Kongsgaard Mads, et al. Human Achilles tendon glycation and function in diabetes. J Appl Physiol 2016;120:130–7.
8. Lamm BM, Gottlieb HD, Paley D. A two-stage percutaneous approach to Charcot diabetic foot reconstruction. J Foot Ankle Surg 2010;49:517–22.
9. Sohn Min-Woong, Stuck Rodney, Pinzur Michael, et al. Lower-extremity amputation risk after Charcot arthropathy and diabetic foot ulcer. Diabetes Care 2010;33(1):98–100.
10. Cherkashin Alexander, Samchukov Mikhail, Birkholts Franz. Treatment Strategies and Frame Configurations in the Management of Foot and Ankle Deformities. Clinics in Podiatric Medicine and surgery 2018;35(4):423–42. https://doi.org/10.1016/j.cpm.2018.05.003.
11. Smith WB, Moore CA. A proposed treatment algorithm for midfoot Charcot arthropathy. Foot and Ankle Specialist 2012;5(1):80–4.
12. Bevilacqua NJ, Rogers LC. Surgical management of Charcot midfoot deformities. Clin Podiatr Med Surg 2008;25:81–94.
13. Schweinberger MH, Roukis TS. Surgical correction of soft-tissue ankle equinus contracture. Clin Podiatr Med Surg 2008;25(4):571–85.

14. Conway JD. Charcot salvage of the foot and ankle using external fixation. Foot Ankle Clin N Am 2008;13:157–73.
15. Roukis TS, Zgonis T. Management of acute Charcot fracture-dislocations with the Taylor's Spatial external fixation system. Clin Podiatr Med Surg 2006;23:467–83.
16. Taylor JC. Six-axis deformity analysis and correction. In: Paley D, editor. Principles of deformity correction. Berlin: Springer-Verlag; 2002. p. 411–36.
17. Siddiqui NA, Pless A. Midfoot and hindfoot Charcot joint deformity correction with hexapod-assisted circular external fixation. Clin Surg 2017;2:1–6.
18. Short DJ, Zgonis T. Management of osteomyelitis and bone loss in the diabetic Charcot foot and ankle. Clin Podiatr Med Surg 2017;34(3):381–7.
19. Sammarco VJ. Superconstructs in Charcot foot deformity. Foot Ankle Clin N Am 2009;14:393–407.
20. Crim Brandon, Lowery Nicholas, Wukich Dane., Internal fixation techniques for midfoot charcot neuroarthropathy in patient with diabetes, *Clin Podiatr Med Surg,* 28, 2011 673–685.
21. Lamm Bradley, Siddiqui Noman, Nair Ajitha, Intramedullary foot fixation for midfoot Charcot Neuroarthropathy, *J Foot Ankle Surg*, 51, 2012, 531-536.
22. Pope Ernest, Takemoto Richelle, Kummer Frederick J, et al. Midfoot fusion: a biomechanical comparison of plantar plating vs intramedullary screws. FAI 2013;34(3):409–13.
23. LaFontaine Javier, Shibuya Naohiro, Sampson Wayne, et al. Trabecular quality and cellular characteristics of normal, diabetic, and Charcot bone. J Foot Ankle Surg 2011;50(6):648–53.
24. Stapleton John, Zgonis Thomas. Surgical reconstruction of the diabetic charcot foot. Clin Podiatr Med Surg 2012;29:425–33.
25. Cullen Benjamin, Weinraub Glenn, Van Gompel Gabriel. Early results with use of the midfoot fusion bolt in Charcot neuroarthropathy. J Foot Ankle Surg 2013;52: 235–8.
26. Sammarco V James, Sammarco G James, Walker Earl, et al. Midtarsal arthrodesis in the treatment of Charcot midfoot arthropathy. JBJS Am 2009;91:80–91.
27. Wiewiorski Martin, Yasui Tetsuro, Miska Matthias, et al. Solid bolt fixation of the medial column in Charcot midfoot arthropathy. J Foot Ankle Surg 2013;52(1): 88–94.
28. Loredo Rebecca, Rahal Andres, Garcia Glenn, et al. Imaging of the diabetic foot: diagnostic dilemmas. Foot and Ankle Specialist 2010;3(5):249–64.
29. Palestro Christopher, Love Charito, Tronco Gene, et al. Combined labeled leukocyte and technetium 99m sulfur colloid bone marrow imaging for diagnosis musculoskeletal infection. RadioGraphics 2006;26(3):859–70.
30. Panagopoulous Periklis, Drosos Georgios, Maltezos Efstratios, et al. Local antibiotic delivery systems in diabetic foot osteomyelitis: time for one step beyond? Int J Lower Extremity Wounds 2015;14(1):87–91.
31. Tsourvakas S. Local antibiotic therapy in the treatment of bone and soft tissue infections. In: Danilla S, editor. Selected topics in reconstructive plastic surgery. Croatia: InTech Europe; 2012. p. 17–44.

Circular Fixation in Charcot

Byron Hutchinson, DPM

KEYWORDS

- Circular fixation • Charcot reconstruction • Charcot foot and ankle

KEY POINTS

- Understanding frame biomechanics during the application of the frame will lead to less complications.
- Prebuilt static frames can decrease time in the operating room and increase efficiency.
- Circular fixation in Charcot foot and ankle deformities improve on the superconstruct concept.

INTRODUCTION

Managing Charcot deformity of the foot and ankle can be very challenging. Part of that challenge is that every case is unique and the timing for optimizing the patient for surgery can be difficult. Although there is agreement that reconstructive surgical intervention can improve the quality of life in these patients and prevent amputation, there is no consensus on the optimal method of reconstruction.[1–3]

The evolution of Charcot reconstruction has moved away from exostectomy in favor of arthrodesis procedures to stabilize the foot and ankle.[4] The goal is to have a plantigrade foot and/or a stable hind foot and ankle, which is free of infection. This goal is accomplished by reduction of the deformity through adequate resection of bone, improving alignment, and then performing fusions that extend beyond the zone of injury.[5–10] The reconstruction requires the use of the strongest implants that the soft tissues will tolerate to maximize the potential for a good outcome. The implants used today in both midfoot and ankle Charcot center around beaming with intramedullary nails, plates, or combinations.

Circular fixation has played a significant role in the management of Charcot foot and ankle over the past 2 decades.[11–16] In the presence of infection or large segmental bone loss with Charcot deformity, circular fixation has been the gold standard.[17,18]

Recently, internal fixation has been combined with circular fixation to achieve successful limb preservation.[19–21]

CHI/Franciscan Advanced Foot & Ankle Fellowship, Franciscan Foot & Ankle Associates: Highline Clinic (Part of Franciscan Medical Group), 16233 Sylvester Road SW G-10, Seattle, WA 98166, USA
E-mail address: highlinef@aol.com

Clin Podiatr Med Surg 39 (2022) 643–658
https://doi.org/10.1016/j.cpm.2022.05.008
0891-8422/22/© 2022 Elsevier Inc. All rights reserved.

This article focuses on the application and indications for static circular fixation in diabetic Charcot disease. The indications for external fixation are listed in **Box 1**.

External fixation in Charcot deformity can be a versatile and powerful tool to reduce deformity gradually or in an acute setting. For example, gradual correction through the use of a Hexapod can help realign the foot in a bayonet deformity, spare the soft tissues, and make the job of definitive arthrodesis more efficient[22–24] (**Figs. 1** and **2**).

Combined internal and external fixation has gained popularity as a new supercon-struct in midfoot and ankle Charcot for many reasons (**Box 2**).

Circular fixation can "protect" the internal fixation by neutralizing the torque and bending forces around the foot and ankle. Circular fixation can be used in patients who cannot stay off their foot and as a device to off-load wounds or soft tissue transfers. In addition, it has been shown that there is synergy between beams and the application of bent wire technique from the foot plate.[25]

APPLICATION OF/AND FRAME BIOMECHANICS

The application of a static circular fixator in Charcot deformities requires an under-standing of frame biomechanics to reduce the possibility of premature removal of the frame, which in turn can compromise the outcome. It is the author's opinion that surgeon's with a lot of experience with the application of circular fixators can apply a suboptimal frame. An orthogonal frame with attention to detail between the bone segments, wires, and half pins is essential. The following discussion is based on available evidence and personal experience.

When possible, having the static frame prebuilt saves a lot of time in the operating room. Smaller-diameter rings have been shown to be more stable than larger rings so that the stability of the frame is impacted the closer the ring is to the bone segment.[26–28] Measuring the circumference of the calf before surgery is helpful in achieving that goal (**Fig. 3**).

The author prefers to have a double proximal tibial ring block to allow for several points of fixation (especially in diabetic Charcot) and is much more stable than one ring with a half pin or a drop wire (**Fig. 4**).

Keeping away from the midtibial area will decrease the chance of tibial fractures, and it also gives one the room for intramedullary nail placement of the desired length because one does not have to worry about the wires and/or half pin proximity to the nail; this of course might be modified if one is doing a distal tibial lengthening where

---

Box 1
Indications for static circular fixation in Charcot

Osteomyelitis (acute and chronic)

Off-loading wounds

Supplement internal fixation

Deformity correction

Lengthen over a nail

Soft tissue coverage

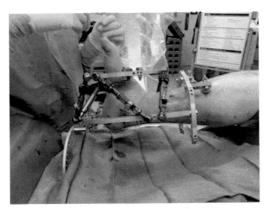

Fig. 1. Butt frame for gradual correction of bayonet deformity.

one might want a tibial ring closer to the corticotomy (see chapter # 11 in this issue). The distal tibial ring should be just above the ankle joint with enough room to accommodate the anterior ankle anatomy.

Connection of the proximal to the distal tibial ring is accomplished with threaded rods, telescoping rods, or rapid adjust struts. Typically, the author uses rapid adjust struts to funnel or cone the frame to allow for variations in the soft tissues from proximal to distal; this helps to keep the distance of the ring to the bone segment as close as possible (**Fig. 5**).

Initially, the placement of connection rods anterior and posterior can be used as an orthogonal guide to align the frame parallel to the tibial crest. In addition, this provides more room for wire and half pin placement. Adding the additional connection rods at the end makes it a lot easier to apply the frame (**Fig. 6**).

The initial attachment of the foot plate to the distal tibial ring is done in a similar fashion with 2 posterior connection rods leaving the rest of the foot plate empty for wire placement and then at the end attaching additional rods (see **Fig. 6**). Placement of the foot plate should be above the plantar aspect of the foot. Generally, the author

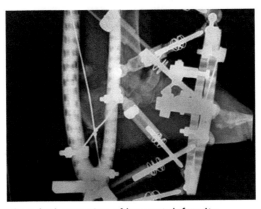

Fig. 2. Radiograph of gradual correction of bayonet deformity.

> **Box 2**
> **Benefits of static circular fixation in Charcot**
>
> Compromised soft tissue envelope
>
> Protect internal fixation "new superconstruct"
>
> Neutralize torque and bending forces
>
> Assumption of weight-bearing
>
> Allows for off-loading of plantar flap or ulcer
>
> Dynamic adjustments can be made
>
> Synergy of bent wire technique with beams

has 3 standard frames for Charcot reconstructions, and they all have the extended proximal tibial double ring block to avoid the midshaft of the tibia and to increase stability to the overall frame construct.

The first frame construct is used for talocalcaneal (TC)/ tibiotalocalcaneal (TTC) fusions with or without internal fixation (**Fig. 7**).

The frame allows for good compression for a TC/TTC fusion. The distal tibial plafond is wider than the shaft of the tibia, and placement of the distal tibial ring in this area makes it easier to pass wire fixation around an intramedullary (IM) nail or lateral plate than in the proximal tibial midshaft.

The second frame allows for compression for a TC fusion in conjunction with a distal tibial lengthening (**Fig. 8**). This construct can also be used for a lengthening over a nail or lengthening and then nailing.

The third frame is for midfoot deformities and can also be used in conjunction with plates or IM beams within the midfoot (**Fig. 9**).

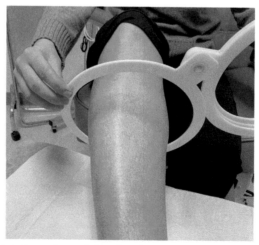

Fig. 3. Sizing template for estimated ring size done preoperatively.

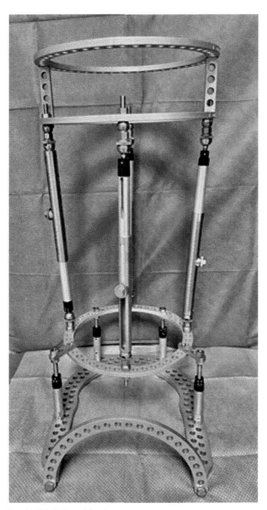

Fig. 4. Double proximal tibial ring block.

Initial alignment of the circular fixator is very important to not only accommodate soft tissue but also have a biomechanically sound construct. Referencing the frame to the bone segment is a critical step to ensure that the frame is orthogonal and in the correct position allowing the surgeon to apply the wires and pins properly depending on the type of deformity that the circular fixation is being applied to manage. The transverse reference wire in the calcaneus is placed first allowing the foot plate to be in a perfect position. Often when the frame is referenced more proximally the foot plate may not be in an ideal place. By placing this pin first, one avoids getting the frame too close to the heel. The second reference wire is placed in the proximal tibial ring. Once the frame is orthogonal in all 3 body planes the rest of the fixation elements can be applied. A knee holder and kickstand can be helpful to elevate the leg, which allows for better delivery of wires and pins; it also makes the use of fluoroscopy easier because the leg is above the opposite leg[29] (**Fig. 10**).

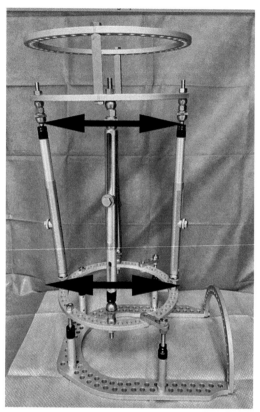

Fig. 5. Using adjustable struts to funnel (cone) the frame to accommodate soft tissues in the lower leg.

Wires and half pins can be applied in a standard sequential fashion for efficiency. Starting with the proximal tibial ring block, a 4-mm half pin is placed bicortical along the tibial face; this is supplemented with a smooth wire, and then this wire is tensioned to 120 kg. This process is repeated in the second tibial ring block. The author recommends using 4-mm half pins. This recommendation is based on biomechanical studies that have shown that 4-mm half pins can allow micromotion equivalent to 2 crossed wires tensioned at 90 kg (**Fig. 11**).[30]

Fixation with olive wires is then performed in the distal tibial ring. These wires are simultaneously tensioned to 120 to 130 kg. The ideal wire angle is hard to achieve, so by simultaneously tensioning the wires there is no loss of tension to the wires and the ring is balanced[30] (**Fig. 12**).

The olives help to prevent any translation of the bone segment in the ring.[31] In addition, there is more bone within the distal tibial ring to accept wires especially when using the circular fixation in conjunction with an IM nail. Additional fixation at each ring can be added especially in the diabetic population to plan for wires and pins that may need to be removed over time. The additional struts can now be added for stability, and this completes the tibial block.

Drawing attention to the foot plate, olive wires are typically used in the calcaneus and midfoot to avoid translation of the foot within the foot plate. The 2 crossed olive

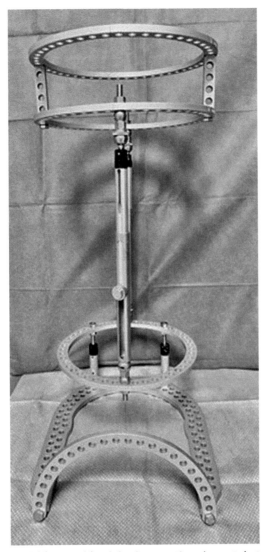

Fig. 6. Showing the initial frame with minimal connection elements between rings and also the foot plate. Additional struts are added once wires and half pins have been placed.

wires are placed in the calcaneus first but not tensioned. Next, the midfoot wires are placed but not tensioned. It is recommended to avoid the metatarsal wires in the diabetic population because they are always at risk of getting infected or breaking. In addition, if the frame is being used in conjunction with beaming, it is difficult to place wires in the metatarsals as well. Additional wires can be attached to the foot plate and bent wire technique along with the beams for compression synergy.[25] In TC fusions, bent wire technique can also be used to fixate the head of talus to the tibia. Samchukov and colleagues[31] have shown that the foot support is mechanically similar to a drop wire construct, with the forefoot wires behaving as the dropped wire. So simultaneously tensioning the forefoot wires to 130 kg and then simultaneously tensioning

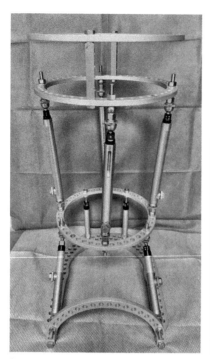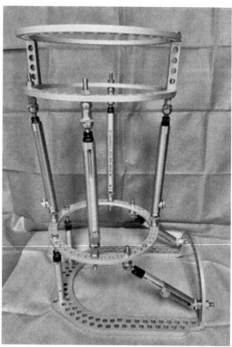

Fig. 7. Circular frame construct for TC/TTC arthrodesis with or without internal fixation.

the calcaneal wires to 90 kg deforms the ring enough to drop tension in the forefoot to exactly 90 kg balancing the frame. This procedure prevents loosening of the calcaneal wires and balances the frame more efficiently.

ANKLE CHARCOT

The vast majority of patients with ankle Charcot cannot be braced because of the severe frontal plane deformity that exists. Therefore, surgical reconstruction for limb preservation is most often the best option. The condition of the soft tissue envelope and the presence or absence of the talus are key considerations in planning in Charcot ankle reconstruction.

If the talus is absent or cannot be used in the reconstruction and a TC fusion is planned, the design of the circular fixator needs to take into consideration whether or not a distal or proximal lengthening is going to be performed along with the primary TC fusion. There are several advantages in doing a distal tibial lengthening in this population of patients. When there is no talus and a primary TC fusion is performed, a distal tibial corticotomy provides for the loss of length, and it has been demonstrated that a corticotomy will increase blood flow at the distal fusion site.[32,33] An IM nail may be used during the index surgery or when the frame is removed for definitive fixation. Solid fusion in the Charcot population is ideal but difficult to accomplish in most cases. Dynamization of the frame and/or IM nail may also be an important factor in improving the chances for solid fusion. The surgeon can plan for dynamization from the beginning by applying modular dynamization devices or attaching these at some point during the rehabilitation process. Current generation IM nails also have the capability to dynamize immediately or at a later date.

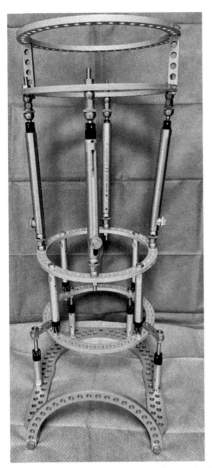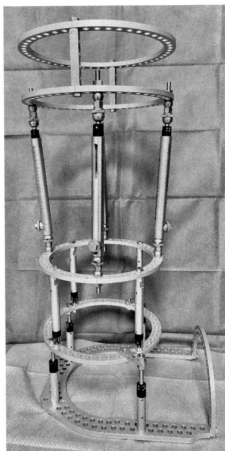

Fig. 8. Circular frame construct for TC fusion with lengthening.

MIDFOOT CHARCOT

Patients who present with midfoot disease respond much better to conventional conservative care options than those with ankle Charcot. The pathomechanics of midfoot disease is highlighted by the presence of equinus, and this creates a compression/tension load on the medial and lateral columns in the foot that is different than the axial load occurring in ankle Charcot. Beaming techniques have been developed to deal with the unique loading forces in midfoot Charcot reconstruction.[9,24,34,35] Circular fixation is often used in conjunction with internal fixation in midfoot Charcot reconstructions.[19,24]

It is important that all joints are prepared and that the hind foot and ankle are reduced before midfoot fixation (**Figs. 13–15**). Relocation of the cuboid and establishment of Meary's angle are imperative. Both columns should be locked with the beams and/or plates being used, and the hind foot should be neutral. The author recommends closing all surgical sites before the application of the prebuilt static frame. Placement of the midfoot wires can be a challenge especially when plates are used.

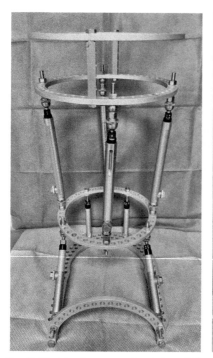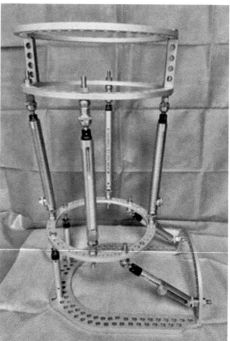

Fig. 9. Circular frame construct for midfoot reconstruction.

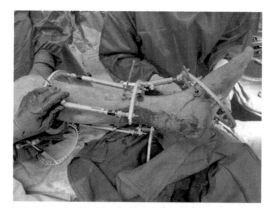

Fig. 10. Note the leg holder under the knee and the "kickstand" distally in this modified flap frame for a hemisoleus muscle flap. The leg is resting higher than the contralateral leg so there is easy access for fluoroscopy and placing wires and pins.

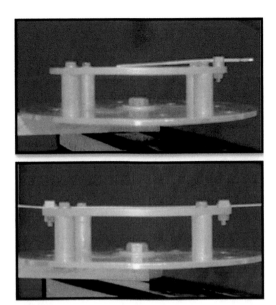

Fig. 11. Axial load of 2 crossed wires at 90-kg tension is equivalent to a 4-mm half pin.

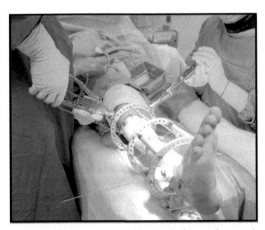

Fig. 12. Simultaneous tensioning on a ring helps to balance the tension regardless of the wire angle.

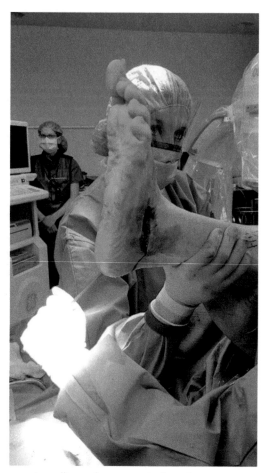

Fig. 13. Note Steinman pin pulling calcaneus out of equinus.

SUMMARY

Circular fixators are extremely versatile in treating Charcot foot and ankle. Dynamic adjustments can be made over time and the frame provides stability to reconstructions in this difficult population. Circular fixation in Charcot can be used to supplement internal fixation or to help stabilize soft tissue coverage such as flaps and grafts. In the presence of osteomyelitis, circular fixation can be used as a primary device with the ability to accommodate large segmental bone defects.

Understanding frame biomechanics is especially important when dealing with Charcot foot and ankle deformities. Prebuilt circular fixators can save time in the operating room and can accommodate most Charcot foot and ankle deformities. Funneling the frame, simultaneous tensioning of wires, and considering tensioning sequence in the foot plate are paramount to successful frame construct and longevity.

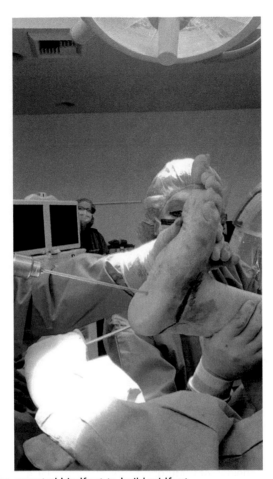

Fig. 14. Pining the corrected hindfoot to build midfoot.

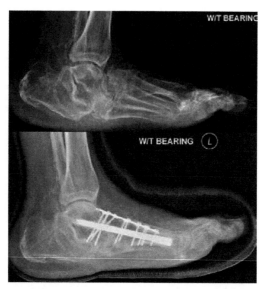

Fig. 15. Note that the midfoot has been built off of a nonreduced hind foot.w

DISCLOSURE

Consultant for Orthofix, Smith & Nephew, Paragon 28, and Metlogix.

REFERENCES

1. Ha Joon, Hester T, Foley R, et al. Charcot foot reconstruction outcomes: a systematic review. J Clin Orhop Trauma 2020;11(3):357–68.
2. Zgonis T, Roukis TS, Lamm BM. Charcot foot and ankle reconstruction: current thinking and surgical approaches. Clin Podiatr Med Sure 2007;24:505.
3. Harkin EA, Schneider AM, Murphy M, et al. Deformity and clinical outcomes following operative correction of Charcot ankle. Foot Ankle Int 2019;40–145.
4. Catanzariti AR, Mendicino R, Haverstock B. Ostectomy for diabetic neuroarthropathy involving the midfoot. J Foot Ankle Surg 2000;39(5):291–300.
5. Cianni L, Bocchi MB, Vitello R, et al. Arthrodesis in the Charcot foot: a systematic review. Orthop Rev 2020;12(Suppl 1):8670.
6. Simon SR, Samir TG, Wilson DL, et al. Arthrodesis as an early alternative to nonoperative management of Charcot artthropathwy of the diabetic foot. J Bone Joint Surg Am 2000;82(7):939.
7. Safavi PS, Jupiter DC, Panchbhavi V. A systematic review of current surgical interventions for Charcot Neuroarthropathy of the midfoot. J Foot Ankle Surg 2017; 56(6):1249–52.
8. Caravaggi CM, Sganzaroli AB, Galenda P, et al. Long-term follow-up of tibiocalcaneal arthrodesis in diabetic patients with early chronic Charcot osteoarthropathy. J Foot Ankle Surg 2012;51(4):408–11.
9. Cullen BD, Weinraub GM, Van Gompel G. Early results with use of the midfoot fusion bolt in Charcot arthropathy. J Foot Ankle Surg 2013;52(2):235–8.
10. Pola LD, Volpe A, Varotto D, et al. Use of a retrograde nail for ankle arthrodesis in Charcot neuroarthropathy: a limb salvage procedure. Foot Ankle Int 2007;28(9): 967–70.

11. Cooper PS. Application of external fixation for management of Charcot deformities of the foot and ankle. Foot Ankle Clin 2002;7:207–54.
12. Farber DC, Juliano PJ, Cavanagh PR, et al. Single stage correction with external fixation of the ulcerated foot in individuals with Charcot neuroarthropathy. Foot Ankle Int 2002;23:130–4.
13. Jolly GP, Zgonis T, Polyzois V. External fixation in the management of Charcot neuroarthropathy. Clin Podiatr Med Sure 2003;20:741–56.
14. Herbst SA. External fixation of Charcot arthropathy. Foot Ankle Clin 2004;9(3): 595–609, x.
15. Pinzur MS. The role of ring external fixation in Charcot foot arthropathy. Foot Ankle Clin 2006;11(4):837–47.
16. Conway JD. Charcot salvage of the foot and ankle using external fixation13. Foot & Ankle Clinics; 2008. p. 157–73.
17. Pinzur MS, Gil J, Belamares J. Treatment of osteomyelitis in Charcot foot with single-stage resection of infection, correction of deformity and maintenance with ring fixation. Foot Ankle Intl 2012;33(12):1069–74.
18. Dalla Paola L, Brocco E, Ceddacci T, et al. Limb albagie in Charcot foot and ankle osteomyelitis: combined use single stage/double stage of arthrodesis and external fixation. Foot Ankle Intl 2009;30(11):1065–70.
19. Hegewald KW, Wilder ML, Chappell TM, et al. Combined internal and external fixation for diabetic Charcot reconstruction: a retrospective case series. J Foot Ankle Surg 2016;55(3):619–27.
20. Brandao RA, Weber JS, Larson D, et al. New fixation methods for the treatment of the diabetic foot: beaming, external fixation, and beyond. Clin Podiatr Med Surg 2018;35(1):63–76.
21. Ettinger S, Plaass C, Claassen L, et al. Sugical management of Charcot deformity for the foot and ankle-radiologic outcome after internal/external fixation. J Foot Ankle Surg 2016;55(3):522–8.
22. Siddiqui NA, LaPorta GA. Midfoot Charcot reconstuction. Clin Podiatr Med Surg 2018;35(4):509–20.
23. Roukis TS, Zgonis T. The management of acute Charcot fracture-dislocations with the taylor's spatial external fixation system. Clin Podiatr Med Surg 2006;23(2): 467–93.
24. Lamm BM, Siddiqui NA, Nair AK, et al. Intramedullary foot fixation for midfoot Charcot neuroarthropathy. J Foot Ankle Surg 2012;51(4):531–6.
25. Grant WP, Rubin LG, Pupp GR, et al. Mechanical testing of seven fixation methods for generation of compression across a mid tarsal osteotomy: a comparison of internal and external fixation methods. J Foot Ankle Surg 2007;46(5): 325–35.
26. Ilizarov GA. The Apparatus: components and biomechanical principles of application. In: Green S, editor. Tranosseous osteosynthesis. Theoretical and clinical aspects of the regeneration and growth of tissue. Berlin: Springer-Verlag; 1992. p. 63–136.
27. Duda GN, Kassi JP, Hoffman JE, et al. Mechanical behavior of Ilizarov ring fixators. Effect of frame parameters on stiffness and consequences for clinical use. Unfallchirurg 2000;103(10):839–45.
28. Cross AR, Lewis DD, Murphy ST, et al. Effects of ring diameter and wire tension on the axial biomechanics of four-ring circular external skeletal fixator constructs. Am J Vet Res 2001;62(7):1025–30.
29. Hutchinson BL, McCann K, Kirienko A. The kickstand technique for circular fixator assembly. J Foot Ankle Surg 2010;49(5):504–5.

30. Calhoun JH, Li F, Bauford WL, et al. Rigidity of half-pins for the Ilizarov external fixator. Hosp Joint Dis 1992;52(1):21–6.
31. Samchukov ML, Clifford CE, McCann KM, et al. Biomechanical considerations in foot and ankle circular external fixation: maintenance of wire tension. Clin Podiatr Med Surg 2018;35(4):443–55.
32. Chen Y, Kuang X, Zhou J, et al. Proximal tibial cortex transverse distraction facilitating healing and limb salvage in severe and recalcitrant diabetic foot ulcers. Clin Orthop Relat Res 2020;478(4):836–51.
33. Aronson J. Temporal and spatial increases in blood flow during distraction osteogenisis. Clin Orthop Relat Res 1994;301:124–31.
34. Grant W, Lavin S, Sabo R. Beaming the columns for Charcot diabetic foot reconstruction: a retrospective analysis. J Foot Ankle Surg 2011;50(2):182–9.
35. Ford SE, Cohen BE, Hodges Davis W, et al. Clinical outcomes and complication of midfoot Charcot reconstruction with intramedullary beaming. Foot Ankle Int 2019;40(1):18–23.

Tibial Lengthening and Intramedullary Nail Fixation for Hindfoot Charcot Neuroarthropathy

Kelsey J. Millonig, DPM, MPH, AACFAS[a],*,
Noman A. Siddiqui, DPM, MHA, FACFAS[b,c]

KEYWORDS

- Ankle • arthrodesis • distraction • fixation • fusion • osteogenesis • tibiocalcaneal
- tibiotalocalcaneal

KEY POINTS

- Outcomes of tibiocalcaneal arthrodesis with distal tibial lengthening in neuropathic patients
- Use of distraction osteogensis for improved vascularity in neuropathic patients
- Principles of external and internal fixation in neuropathic patients

INTRODUCTION

Charcot neuroarthropathy is a debilitating condition that impacts patient function and places them at high risk for limb loss. Many patients with Charcot neuroarthropathy experience severe soft tissue deformity and osseous fragmentation. This increases the threat of concurrent osteomyelitis that can further complicate reconstruction scenarios. Charcot neuroarthropathy may be midfoot or hindfoot driven, each requiring different surgical reconstructive approaches. The distribution of Charcot neuroarthropathy involvement varies in the literature; the midfoot is most commonly involved. Schon and colleagues[1] found the anatomic distribution to be 22.6% ankle, 10.0% hindfoot, 59.2% midfoot, and 8.0% forefoot.

The goal of any Charcot surgical reconstruction is to establish a stable plantigrade foot enabling patients to be community ambulators.[2] When correcting these deformities, segmental bone loss may occur because of bone resection for acute reduction

a East Village Foot & Ankle Surgeons, 500 East Court Avenue, Suite 314, Des Moines, IA 50309, USA; b International Center for Limb Lengthening, Rubin Institute for Advanced Orthopedics, Sinai Hospital of Baltimore, Baltimore, MD 21215, USA; c Department of Podiatry, Northwest Hospital, Randallstown, MD 21133, USA
* Corresponding author.
E-mail address: Kelsey.J.Millonig@gmail.com

Clin Podiatr Med Surg 39 (2022) 659–673
https://doi.org/10.1016/j.cpm.2022.05.011
0891-8422/22/© 2022 Elsevier Inc. All rights reserved.

of angular deformity or removal of nonviable avascular bone.[3] This poses a particular challenge in hindfoor or ankle-driven Charcot neuroarthropathy. There is no consensus for improving arthrodesis or managing segmental defects in the neuropathic foot and ankle.

The most viable treatment option for hindfoot or ankle Charcot neuroarthropathy deformity is an arthrodesis of the tibiocalcaneal or tibiotalocalcaneal complex. Fragomen and colleagues[4] reported in their study of complex fusions that patients with Charcot neuroarthropathy had higher rates of nonunion, complications, and subsequent subtalar joint failure. Given the subtalar joint failure, they recommended tibiotalocalcaneal fusion for all Charcot neuroarthropathy cases with ankle pathology.[4] Several surgical techniques are available for these hindfoot/ankle fusions, including intramedullary nail fixation, plating, external fixation, or a combination technique.

There are multiple challenges associated with arthrodesis because hindfoot or ankle Charcot often yields avascular necrosis or chronic dislocation of the talus with nonviable bone (**Fig. 1**). Alternative treatments such as bone grafting techniques may not be viable, available, or are contraindicated. There is a necessity to find effective alternatives to assist with achieving arthrodesis in these patients. It has been well established in the literature that the biologic effects of Charcot neuroarthropathy on osseous structures make arthrodesis difficult to obtain, resulting in infection, malunion, or nonunion, thereby keeping the patient at risk for limb loss. Histologic reports demonstrate that Charcot neuroarthropathy bone has a disorganized trabecular pattern and is infiltrated with inflammatory myxoid tissue, presumptively indicating why nonunions are encountered frequently.[5] Time to arthrodesis is often prolonged, requiring extended periods of nonweightbearing. Identifying successful techniques for Charcot neuroarthropathy is imperative in a population with high nonunion rate for tibiotalocalcaneal and tibiocalcaneal fusion.

Arthrodesis rates reported with exclusive use of circular external fixation for Charcot neuroarthropathy have an extensive range, including 50% (n = 12), 90% at a mean 4 months (n = 11), and 86% with circular external fixation in place for fusion for a

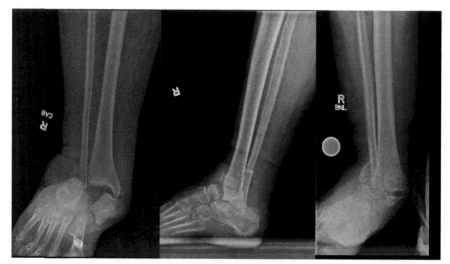

Fig. 1. Patient with Charcot neuroarthropathy demonstrating chronic dislocation of the talus yielding nonviable bone. Copyright 2020, Rubin Institute for Advanced Orthopedics, Sinai Hospital of Baltimore, used with permission.

mean of 6.5 months (n = 45).[6–8] The exclusive use of a retrograde intramedullary nail for ankle arthrodesis presented an osseous arthrodesis rate of 77.7% (n = 18).[9] Yammine and Assi[10] completed a meta-analysis comparing these techniques observing weighted fusion rates of 74% for circular external fixation with mean time to radiographic union of 8.5 months and 90.7% for intramedullary nailing with a mean time to arthrodesis of 7.3 months. Both techniques are frequently used, but show varying results.

PRESENCE OF WOUND/INFECTION

The presence of infection significantly impacts the treatment approach. It is the opinion of the authors that in the presence of a wound, infection should be evaluated with preoperative laboratory values and a staged approach should be used. The initial phase should consider excision of the wound, removal of hardware if present, deep intraoperative soft tissue and bone cultures, and removal of all nonviable tissue and bone (**Fig. 2**). If osteomyelitis is diagnosed, an antibiotic-impregnated polymethylmethacrylate spacer with vancomycin and tobramycin is placed locally and systemic intravenous antibiotics should be used, based on cultures (**Fig. 3**).

DISTRACTION OSTEOGENESIS YIELDING HYPERVASCULARIZATION

Distraction osteogenesis with circular external fixation has been reported for use in osseous defects with hindfoot deformity or complicated ankle arthrodesis.[11] As Ilizarov originally hypothesized, distraction osteogenesis yields a hypervascular environment to the osteotomy or corticotomy site and adjacent joint arthrodesis, potentially accelerating fusion of the ankle arthrodesis and assisting in the control of any present infection. Measured blood flow during distraction osteogenesis with quantitative technetium scintigraphy has demonstrated a two- to three-fold increase in blood flow compared with the contralateral site.[12] There has been examples in

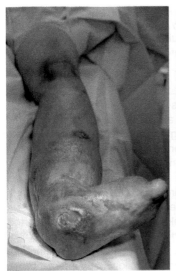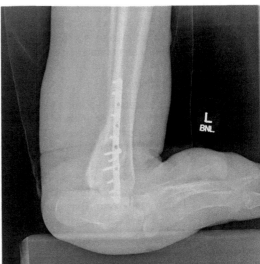

Fig. 2. Patient presents with significant lower extremity wound that requires staging operative procedures. Copyright 2020, Rubin Institute for Advanced Orthopedics, Sinai Hospital of Baltimore, used with permission.

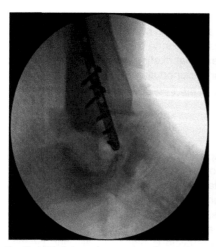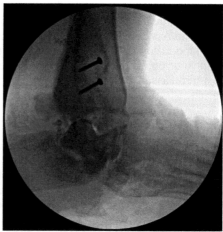

Fig. 3. Initial staged procedure for patient with chronic wound requiring intraoperative cultures, hardware removal, and placement of localized antibiotic spacer. Copyright 2020, Rubin Institute for Advanced Orthopedics, Sinai Hospital of Baltimore, used with permission.

animal tibial models of vascular proliferation occurring actively during the latency and distraction periods and then gradually decreasing over time.[13] Additionally, close temporal and spatial relationships exist between formation of regenerate bone and vascular proliferation of the periosteum and medullary canal.[13] An animal study reported that vascular flow at the distraction site increased 10 times compared with the control at 2 weeks postdistraction osteogenesis. The distraction site then decreased to four to five times the control for the remainder of the distraction period. Continuing through the consolidation phase, vascular flow continued to be two to three times the control. Prolonged hypervascularization was also demonstrated distally in the tibia, but at a decreased ratio to the proximal distraction osteogenesis site, ranging from 1.6 to 5 times less.[14] Additionally, the rate of distraction osteogenesis has also been described to increase the vascularization process with the central fibrous zone maximally stimulated at distraction rates of 0.7 and 1.3 mm/d.[15]

Proximal Tibial Lengthening

There is a paucity of literature reporting the benefits of distraction osteogenesis in the setting of a complex hindfoot or ankle arthrodesis, and even less with specific regard for Charcot neuroarthropathy. Proximal tibial lengthenings are frequently used for tibial lengthening. Fragomen and colleagues[4] reported on complex ankle fusion, detailing that 24 of 91 (26.3%) patients underwent proximal tibial lengthening to normalize limb length several weeks after index arthrodesis had been achieved, excluding tibiocalcaneal and tibiotalocalcaneal arthrodesis. The proximal tibial lengthening yielded an 83% union rate. Their study included 15 patients with Charcot neuroarthropathy, of which 73% achieved union at the ankle; however, it was not reported if any of those patients underwent distraction osteogenesis. Lou and colleagues[16] obtained fusion in all 12 patients in their case series with simultaneous proximal tibial distraction osteogenesis and complex ankle arthrodesis, followed by internal fixation with plating. However, they excluded patients with peripheral neuropathy or severe neurovascular compromise. Tellisi and colleagues[17] reported on 10 of 12 (83.3%) patients undergoing a tibiocalcaneal fusion with a simultaneous proximal tibial lengthening. Mean external fixation time was 8.4 months; all osteotomy sites healed and bone union was achieved in 84% of cases at the initial attempt.

Distal Tibial Lengthening

Distal tibial lengthening with complex arthrodesis is significantly less studied. Chappell and colleagues[11] evaluated distal tibial distraction osteogenesis in various pathologies; of four patients who underwent tibiocalcaneal arthrodesis with distal tibial distraction osteogenesis, three patients (75%) underwent fusion, and one patient (25%) experienced an infected nonunion. When analyzing the literature, no comparative study was found of tibiocalcaneal or tibiotalocalcaneal arthrodesis with distal tibial distraction osteogenesis via circular external fixation in patients with Charcot neuroarthropathy.

The authors prefer a technique using distraction osteogenesis in the distal tibia and circular external fixation, and assert that it improves the adjacent tibiocalcaneal or tibiotalocalcaneal arthrodesis rates in the neuropathic patient. In our own study, 15 patients with a diagnosis of Charcot neuroarthropathy and ankle-level deformity underwent this technique.[18] Mean follow-up from index procedure was 17.5 ± 5.5 months, with 2 to 3 months between circular external fixation application and removal. Radiographic union rate was 93.3% for tibiocalcaneal or tibiotalocalcaneal arthrodesis. Mean time to tibiocalcaneal or tibiotalocalcaneal arthrodesis was 4.75 ± 3.4 months, with most demonstrating union at time of external fixation removal at 3.1 months. One patient had a stable asymptomatic hypertrophic nonunion at last follow-up visit (15 months post index procedure).

A radiographic union scale used in tibial (RUST) fractures score that has shown high reliability was modified to assess successful maturation of the regenerate.[19] A RUST score of 12 is assigned to the regenerate when each of the four cortices demonstrates no visible lucency with the presence of bone callus formation, also known as a RUST score of 3 per cortex. A RUST score of 12 was achieved at the regenerate site at a rate of 86.7%. Three cortices were present at a mean of 6.2 ± 2.2 months, and a RUST score of 12 was achieved in the regenerate at 9.8 ± 3.3 months. Two patients had stable asymptomatic hypertrophic nonunions at the regenerate site at 13 months follow-up visits, respectively. These have not required any treatment because they are asymptomatic hypertrophic nonunions, stable with intramedullary fixation, and continue to demonstrate improved callus formation with serial radiographs.

These concepts regarding hypervascularization and proximity are significant and pertain to the surgical technique discussed next. First, simultaneous distraction osteogenesis and arthrodesis during the initial fusion procedure benefits the arthrodesis site by enabling the highest increase in blood flow during latency and the distraction period. If the procedures are staged, the benefit of the initial hypervascular environment is lost. This is exemplified in this clinical figure of a patient who had substantial hair growth of the lower extremity during osteogenesis (**Fig. 4**). Second, a distal tibial corticotomy, compared with a more proximal tibial osteotomy, spatially places the distraction osteogenesis and fusion sites within close proximity. Therefore, the arthrodesis site benefits to a greater extent through vascular proliferation and prolonged hypervascularization at the distal site. Third, the distraction rate, especially in patients with comorbidities, such as Charcot neuroarthropathy, is important to optimize for vascular proliferation.

Surgical Technique

The articular surfaces of the distal tibia and subtalar joint are removed. The anterior and posterior tibial plafond bone are resected in a manner to create a "cuplike" fit

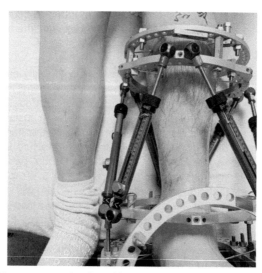

Fig. 4. Substantial improvement in clinical hair growth on the limb undergoing distraction osteogenesis as compared with the contralateral limb suggesting improvement in vascularity. Copyright 2020, Rubin Institute for Advanced Orthopedics, Sinai Hospital of Baltimore, used with permission.

into the anterior aspect of the calcaneus. The tibiotalocalcaneal and tibiocalcaneal complex is fixated with a circular external fixation. There are several external fixation constructs that may be used; the authors prefer a tibial block with two tibial rings proximal and one tibial ring distal to the corticotomy site. It is imperative that the foot external fixation block be acutely compressed 5 to 8 mm with axial-threaded rods fixed across the fusion site to the distal tibial block. This is best attained when the foot plate is placed as close as possible to the distal tibial block, allowing for controlled compression across the arthrodesis site.

The osteotomy for distraction osteogenesis is performed just proximal to the arthrodesis at the metaphyseal diaphyseal junction of the distal tibia. In the author's experience of 15 patients, mean distance was 4.6 cm from the arthrodesis site (**Fig. 5**). There are several options for making the osteotomy including percutaneous or miniopen incisions with a multiple drill-hole technique (**Figs. 6** and **7**). The tibial rings on either side of the corticotomy are connected with six-axis multiplanar struts allowing for distraction osteogenesis at the distal tibial corticotomy site (**Fig. 8**). We contend that patients with Charcot neuroarthropathy should have the opportunity to partially weightbear on their external fixators, given the high-risk nature of these patients with numerous comorbidities and difficulty with nonweightbearing compliance. This is accomplished with an external fixator construct with either a plantar floating ring or rocker bottom (**Fig. 9**).

Postoperative Protocol

Latency period must be considered for any lengthening. The timeframe should be based on the patient's specific conditions and potentially extended due to comorbidities that may delay healing. The mean latency period in the authors' experience with distal tibial lengthening in neuropathic patients is 19.1 $\pm$ 5.5 days with a distraction period of 36.2 $\pm$ 14.6 days. The rate of distraction should be slowed in Charcot

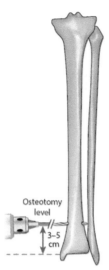

Fig. 5. Illustration of distal tibial osteotomy level. Copyright 2020, Rubin Institute for Advanced Orthopedics, Sinai Hospital of Baltimore, used with permission.

neuroarthropathy patients; the authors used a rate of 0.7 mm/d. Serial radiographs should be obtained during the postoperative phase to monitor regenerate formation, consolidation, and arthrodesis (**Fig. 10**). External fixation is removed when the desired limb length is achieved and regenerate is visible in anteroposterior and lateral radiographic views. The stability of the regenerate and arthrodesis site should always be tested intraoperatively.

COMBINED INTERNAL FIXATION WITH EXTERNAL FIXATION

It is the surgeon's discretion to use this technique with external fixation only or also use an intramedullary nail for additional internal fixation. Two options for timing of intramedullary fixation follow next. Patients are placed in a short leg cast for 2 to 4 weeks after external fixation removal. At the first follow-up appointment after frame removal, the

Pattern for performing minimally invasive
multiple drill-hole osteotomy

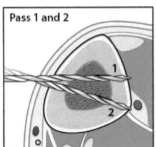

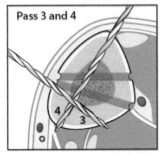

Fig. 6. Pattern to perform minimally invasive drill-hole osteotomy. Copyright 2020, Rubin Institute for Advanced Orthopedics, Sinai Hospital of Baltimore, used with permission.

Two options for completing the osteotomy

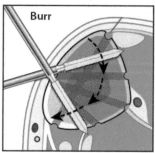 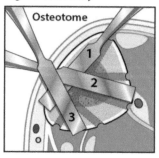

Fig. 7. Options to complete the osteotomy with minimally invasive burr or osteotome. Copyright 2020, Rubin Institute for Advanced Orthopedics, Sinai Hospital of Baltimore, used with permission.

authors recommend that the patients can begin weightbearing in a walking boot with an assistive device.

Combining arthrodesis with distraction osteogenesis often requires retention of the external fixator for longer periods of time, which may enhance the risk of pin-tract infections, loosening of the device, and psychological stress. However, circular external fixation offers benefits, such as the ability to debride radically all infection or poor-quality bone; providing stability in different planes; allowing dynamic axial

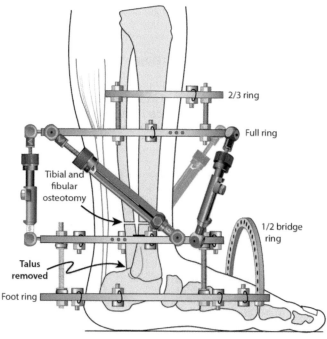

Fig. 8. Illustration of external fixation construction with completed osteotomy after tibiocalcaneal arthrodesis from lateral view. Copyright 2020, Rubin Institute for Advanced Orthopedics, Sinai Hospital of Baltimore, used with permission.

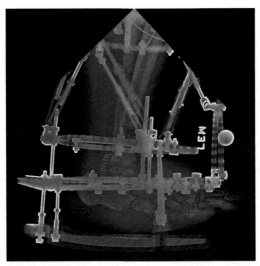

Fig. 9. External fixation construction for distraction osteogenesis with demonstrated rocker rails for ambulation. Copyright 2020, Rubin Institute for Advanced Orthopedics, Sinai Hospital of Baltimore, used with permission.

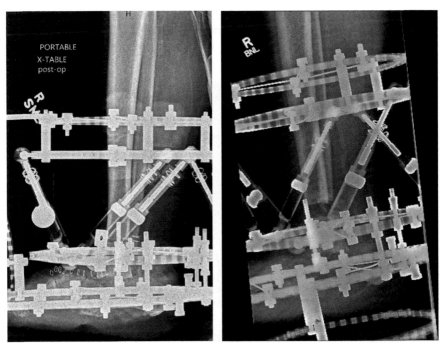

Fig. 10. Serial radiographs demonstrating initial corticotomy and evaluating the distraction site during lengthening. Copyright 2020, Rubin Institute for Advanced Orthopedics, Sinai Hospital of Baltimore, used with permission.

compression at the arthrodesis site, which enhances healing; and enabling distraction osteogenesis.[16]

The pros and cons of using internal fixation combined or staged with external fixation have been long debated. Intramedullary nailing has been suggested to have positive biologic effects on bone healing. These include compensatory increase of periosteal circulation, stimulating periosteal bone formation, and blood flow in the cortex returning to normal and even supernormal levels within days after medullary reaming. Additionally, there is increased osteoinductivity through the local bone graft effect of reamed debris and activation of growth factors and inflammatory responses that are helpful for bone formation.[20–22]

Lengthening Over a Nail

Lengthening over a nail (LON) technique also is used where the retrograde intramedullary nail is inserted in standard fashion; however, this is completed at the time of the index procedure. The proximal tibial nail screws are not placed until the time of external fixation removal when distal tibial lengthening has been completed (**Fig. 11**). The benefits of LON have been well-described to assist in appropriate alignment during distraction osteogenesis, prevent deformity during lengthening, and reduce the risk of refracture after frame removal compared with the classic Ilizarov method.[21] However, some studies have suggested that bone healing time seems to be longer than the classic circular external fixation technique, because it may limit endosteal circulation and increase risk of deep infection with implant at index procedure concurrent with external fixation pin tracts.[22–24]

Lengthening and Then Nailing Technique

To enable external fixation to be removed despite the regenerate not yet achieving complete consolidation, the lengthening and then nailing (LATN) may be used. A permanent retrograde intramedullary nail is inserted at the time of external fixation

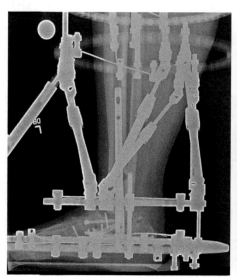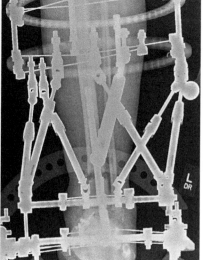

Fig. 11. LON technique demonstrating placement of the intramedullary nail at time of external fixation application with distraction osteogenesis. Copyright 2020, Rubin Institute for Advanced Orthopedics, Sinai Hospital of Baltimore, used with permission.

following lengthening (**Fig. 12**). A guidewire is inserted retrograde through the distal arthrodesis site and into the canal through the distracted callus. The intramedullary nail provides internal stability of the distracted callus and the arthrodesis site, while also maintaining length and alignment and allowing the regenerate bone to mature (**Fig. 13**).

The advantages of the LATN are extensive, including shorter external fixation treatment time, ability to insert a full-length large-diameter nail for more stability, no concomitant use of internal and external fixation reducing risk of infection, flexible timing of intramedullary nail insertion allowing for gradual deformity correction, quicker bone healing, and protection against refracture.[22] In a direct comparison of the two techniques, enhanced bone formation was found with LATN as compared with LON, because of avoiding reaming during the distraction phase, which in turn led to more robust bone regenerate.[21] Another explanation for this effect may be the preservation of endosteal circulation during distraction.[21]

LATN is the authors' preferred method, because it offers the ability to manage infections during distraction osteogenesis with circular external fixation and at time of intramedullary nailing enhance blood flow, provide enhanced stability in these high-risk patients, stabilize the regenerate during consolidation, and allow earlier external fixation removal. LATN is particularly useful in patients with Charcot neuroarthropathy because of their increased risks for infection, nonunion, osseous fragmentation, concurrent peripheral vascular disease, and complication.

The authors suggest using a retrograde femoral intramedullary nail through the calcaneus into the proximal tibia and locked with static screw fixation. A concern with retrograde intramedullary nail fixation is stress risers or fatigue fractures within

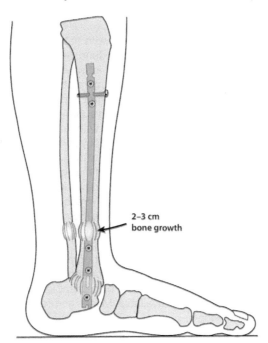

2–3 cm
bone growth

Fig. 12. Intramedullary nail fixation following external fixation removal with callus formation at distraction site and union at tibiocalcaneal arthrodesis site from lateral view. Copyright 2020, Rubin Institute for Advanced Orthopedics, Sinai Hospital of Baltimore, used with permission.

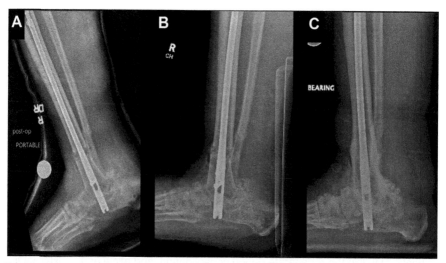

Fig. 13. Charcot neuroarthropathy deformity case with talectomy, tibiocalcaneal fusion with distal tibial distraction osteogenesis in circular external fixation, and then intramedullary nailing with lateral and anteroposterior view radiographs at stages throughout treatment. External fixation removal with intramedullary nail fixation (*A*). Four months after index procedure (*B*). Fifteen months after index procedure (*C*). Copyright 2020, Rubin Institute for Advanced Orthopedics, Sinai Hospital of Baltimore, used with permission.

the tibia. The femoral nail provides the ability for a longer intramedullary nail fixation that extends more proximal than the previous circular external fixation proximal tibial ring where the tibial cortex has been violated with half-pins or wires. The increased length also allows the intramedullary nail to extend beyond the isthmus of the tibia where many of the currently designed hindfoot intramedullary nails end. The authors theorize that these hindfoot nails may result in more stress risers that could yield fatigue fractures from the proximal end of the intramedullary nail, placing increased strain on the tibia in an area of brittle bone. This is supported by a biomechanical study demonstrating that in tibiocalcaneal arthrodesis with retrograde intramedullary nail, a longer nail terminating in the proximal tibial metaphysis reduces the stress concentration, and therefore may be preferred in patients with suboptimal bone.[25]

There is no need to ream the proximal aspect of the tibial metaphysis because of the medullary concentration with widening of the cortex with intramedullary nail insertion and the posterior bend of the femoral nail places stress on the posterior aspect of the tibia. This stress shields the tibia proximally where the strain is placed by the proximal end of the intramedullary nail. The screw fixation of the femoral nail insertion also offers an anteroposterior screw in the dense cortical bone in the tibia proximally, rather than in the cancellous bone in the calcaneus as with retrograde hindfoot intramedullary nail. This is particularly important with Charcot neuroarthropathy because the calcaneus often has poor bone stock, making less ideal placement for screw fixation from anterior to posterior where less cortex is available. Means and colleagues[26,] discussed the importance of a solid anterior-to-posterior oriented screw to prevent sagittal deformation of the arthrodesis site with weightbearing, although they did not look at the exact screw construct discussed in this technique.

The authors have seen intraoperatively that the bend of the femoral nail inserted retrograde allows improved positioning of the foot (**Fig. 14**), preventing it from moving forward and keeping the appropriate anatomic alignment for tibiocalcaneal or

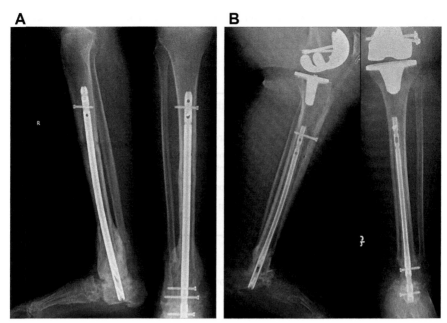

Fig. 14. Lateral and anteroposterior view radiographs of two patients who achieved radiographic union and a RUST score of 12 at the regenerate site. Copyright 2020, Rubin Institute for Advanced Orthopedics, Sinai Hospital of Baltimore, used with permission. (*A*), patient example 1. (*B*), patient example 2.

tibiocalcaneal fusion when markers of normal anatomy are absent, as is often the case with Charcot neuroarthropathy.

MANAGEMENT OF COMPLICATIONS

All surgical reconstruction associated with Charcot neuroarthropathy yields the potential for complications, a fact that has been well reported in the literature. These may include deep infected hardware or external fixation complications requiring modification. Minor complications may also occur, such as continued residual limb length discrepancy requiring a shoe lift, superficial wounds, or pin-site infections. Regarding distal tibial lengthening with tibiocalcaneal or tibiotalocalcaneal arthrodesis, postoperative complications requiring surgical intervention occurred in 3 of 15 patients. Because of the potential for complications, it is imperative that surgeons who use these techniques have an extensive understanding of pathology of Charcot and external fixation.

SUMMARY

Hindfoot and ankle Charcot neuroarthropathy is a challenging condition to treat, specifically with segmental bone defects secondary to avascular necrosis or infection. Several techniques exist alongside continued challenges of nonunion and complication rates. The authors assert that combining distal tibial distraction osteogenesis with external fixation in tibiocalcaneal or tibiotalocalcaneal arthrodesis should be considered an effective method for management of complex Charcot neuroarthropathy conditions of the ankle. This staged procedure technique resulted in a high rate of union in patients who are often considered a high risk for nonunion, and eradication of infection, minimal soft tissue disruption, and improvement in limb length.

CLINICS CARE POINTS

- Simulataneous distraction osteogenesis at the time of hindfoot and ankle arthrodesis is imperative to yield benefits of vascularity.
- Proximity of the coritcotomy site to the arthrodesis site is beneficial for vascularity.
- Distraction rate should be approximately 0.7mm per day and extended latency period due to complex comorbidities in neuropathic patients
- Perform fibular osteotomy at same level to produce synostosis to enhance stability of limb
- Intramedullary nailing will reduce time in external fixation and protect neuropathic regenerate during consolidation.

ACKNOWLEDGMENT

The authors thank Robert P. Farley, BS, for his assistance with this manuscript.

DISCLOSURES

K.J. Millonig is a Consultant for Orthofix. N.A. Siddiqui is a consultant for Arthrex. The following organizations supported the institution of NAS: Biocomposites, DePuy Synthes Companies, MHE Coalition, Orthofix, OrthoPediatrics, Pega Medical, Smith+'''Nephew, Stryker, and Zimmer Biomet.

REFERENCES

1. Schon LC, Easley ME, Weinfeld SB. Charcot neuroarthropathy of the foot and ankle. Clin Orthop Relat Res 1998;349:116–31.
2. Siddiqui NA, LaPorta GA. Midfoot Charcot reconstruction. Clin Podiatr Med Surg 2018;35:509–20.
3. Siddiqui NA, Pless A. Midfoot and hindfoot Charcot joint deformity correction with hexapod-assisted circular external fixation. Clin Surg 2017;2:1430.
4. Fragomen AT, Borst E, Schachter L, et al. Complex ankle arthrodesis using the Ilizarov method yields a high rate of fusion. Clin Orthop Relat Res 2012;470: 2864–73.
5. La Fontaine J, Shibuya N, Sampson HW, et al. Trabecular quality and cellular characteristics of normal, diabetic, and Charcot bone. J Foot Ankle Surg 2011; 50:648–53.
6. Fabrin J, Larsen K, Holstein PE. Arthrodesis with external fixation in the unstable or misaligned Charcot ankle in patients with diabetes mellitus. Int J Low Extrem Wounds 2007;6:102–7.
7. Karapinar H, Senar M, Kazimoglu C, et al. Arthrodesis of neuropathic ankle joint by Ilizarov fixator in diabetic patients. J Am Podiatr Med Assoc 2009;99:42–8.
8. Dalla Paola L, Brocco E, Ceccacci T, et al. Limb salvage in Charcot foot and ankle osteomyelitis: combined use single stage/double stage of arthrodesis and external fixation. Foot Ankle Int 2009;30:1065–76.
9. Dalla Paola L, Volpe A, Varotto D, et al. Use of a retrograde nail for ankle arthrodesis in Charcot neuroarthropathy: a limb salvage procedure. Foot Ankle Int 2007; 28:967–70.

10. Yammine K, Assi C. Intramedullary nail versus external fixator for ankle arthrodesis in Charcot neuroarthropathy: a meta-analysis of comparative studies. J Orthop Surg (Hong Kong) 2019;27(2). 2309499019836012.

11. Chappell TM, Ebert CC, McCann KM, et al. Distal tibial distraction osteogenesis-an alternative approach to addressing limb length discrepancy with concurrent hindfoot and ankle reconstruction. J Orthop Surg Res 2019;14:244.

12. Sakurakichi K, Tsuchiya H, Uehara K, et al. Ankle arthrodesis combined with tibial lengthening using the Ilizarov apparatus. J Orthop Sci 2003;8:20–5.

13. Choi IH, Ahn JH, Chung CY, et al. Vascular proliferation and blood supply during distraction osteogenesis: a scanning electron microscopic observation. J Orthop Res 2000;18:698–705.

14. Aronson J. Temporal and spatial increases in blood flow during distraction osteogenesis. Clin Orthop Relat Res 1994;301:124–31.

15. Li G, Simpson AH, Kenwright J, et al. Effect of lengthening rate on angiogenesis during distraction osteogenesis. J Orthop Res 1999;17:362–7.

16. Lou TF, Hamushan M, Li H, et al. Staged distraction osteogenesis followed by arthrodesis using internal fixation as a form of surgical treatment for complex conditions of the ankle. Bone Joint J 2018;100-B:755–60.

17. Tellisi N, Fragomen AT, Ilizarov S, et al. Limb salvage reconstruction of the ankle with fusion and simultaneous tibial lengthening using the Ilizarov/Taylor spatial frame. HSS J 2008;4:32–42.

18. Siddiqui NA, Millonig KJ, Mayer BE, Fink JN, McClure PK, Bibbo C. Increased arthrodesis rates in Charcot neuroarthropathy utilizing distal tibial distraction osteogenesis principles. Foot Ankle Spec 2022. https://doi.org/10.1177/19386400221087822. PAPed 5/3/22.

19. Azevedo Filho FA, Cotias RB, Azi ML, et al. Reliability of the radiographic union scale in tibial fractures (RUST). Rev Bras Ortop 2016;52:35–9.

20. Danckwardt-Lillieström G. Reaming of the medullary cavity and its effect on diaphyseal bone. A fluorochromic, microangiographic and histologic study on the rabbit tibia and dog femur. Acta Orthop Scand Suppl 1969;128:1–153.

21. Ryu KJ, Kim BH, Hwang JH, et al. Reamed intramedullary nailing has an adverse effect on bone regeneration during the distraction phase in tibial lengthening. Clin Orthop Relat Res 2016;474:816–24.

22. Rozbruch SR, Kleinman D, Fragomen AT, et al. Limb lengthening and then insertion of an intramedullary nail: a case-matched comparison. Clin Orthop Relat Res 2008;466:2923–32.

23. Draenert KD. CORR Insights: reamed intramedullary nailing has an adverse effect on bone regeneration during the distraction phase in tibial lengthening. Clin Orthop Relat Res 2016;474:825–6.

24. Guo Q, Zhang T, Zheng Y, et al. Tibial lengthening over an intramedullary nail in patients with short stature or leg-length discrepancy: a comparative study. Int Orthop 2012;36:179–84.

25. Thordarson DB, Chang D. Stress fractures and tibial cortical hypertrophy after tibiotalocalcaneal arthrodesis with an intramedullary nail. Foot Ankle Int 1999;20:497–500.

26. Means KR, Parks BG, Nguyen A, et al. Intramedullary nail fixation with posterior-to-anterior compared to transverse distal screw placement for tibiotalocalcaneal arthrodesis: a biomechanical investigation. Foot Ankle Int 2006;27:1137–42.

Plate Fixation in Midfoot and Ankle Charcot Neuroarthropathy

Henry D. Spingola III, DPM[a], John Martucci, DPM[a],
Lawrence A. DiDomenico, DPM[a,b,*]

KEYWORDS

- Plate fixation • Midfoot • Ankle • Charcot neuroarthropathy

KEY POINTS

- Healthy resection of diseased bone is necessary/mandatory to provide a healthy environment for bone healing. When the surgeon is attempting a surgical repair, he or she must resect/remove the diseased pathologic bone to good healthy bleeding bone.
- Anatomic alignment should be the goal of the reconstruction. With larger deformities with Charcot reconstruction, it is necessary to achieve a close-to-anatomic alignment with the construct.
- Stable rigid internal fixation is needed for a successful outcome to assist with stabilizing the diseased bone.

INTRODUCTION

Charcot neuroarthropathy (CN) of the foot and ankle is most often observed in the midfoot. Classifications laid out in the early literature began by focusing on broad radiographic findings—development, coalescence, and reconstitution—such as those of Dr Sidney Eichenholtz.[1] Shibata and colleagues recommended a prodromal phase or "stage 0," which is associated with warmth, swelling, and erythema before radiographic changes.[2,3]

Another widely used classification is the Brodsky classification. This system is based on anatomic location affected with types arranged from most common to least commonly identified: type 1, tarsometatarsal joint; type 2, Chopart or subtalar or both; type 3a, ankle; and type 3b, calcaneal tuberosity[1,2] (**Figs. 1–3**).

CN was originally identified by Jean Martin Charcot in patients with peripheral neuropathy from tertiary syphilis. At present, the vast majority of cases are commonly

[a] NOMS Ankle and Foot Care Centers, 8175 Market Street, Youngstown, Ohio 44512, USA;
[b] NOMS Ankle and Foot Care Centers, 16844 Street, Clair Avenue, East Liverpool, Ohio 43920, USA
* Corresponding author. 8175 Market Street, Youngstown, OH 44512.
E-mail address: LD5353@aol.com

Clin Podiatr Med Surg 39 (2022) 675–693
https://doi.org/10.1016/j.cpm.2022.06.001
0891-8422/22/© 2022 Elsevier Inc. All rights reserved.

podiatric.theclinics.com

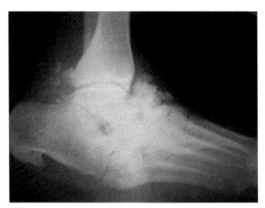

Fig. 1. Radiograph of a diabetic patient who suffers from a midfoot Charcot arthropathy.

associated with long-standing peripheral neuropathy in diabetic patients.[4,5] Although it can be agreed upon that neuropathy is present in the development of CN, diabetes is one comorbidity that stands out in the literature.[5] The association between CN and diabetes was first made by William Riely Jordan in 1936. Since then, given the rise of diabetes, studies highlight its evolution in this population.[4–9] A 5-year retrospective study of 1050 patients revealed 18.8% with diabetes alone died, 28.3% with diabetes and Charcot arthropathy of the foot and/or ankle died, and 37% with diabetes and an ulcer died. The development of an ulcer or CN in a diabetic patient is best thought of as marker of severe disease rather than precursor to demise.[7]

The clinician and surgeon should be aware of the many other causes of peripheral neuropathy that can propagate Charcot joint disease, including disorders such as idiopathic sensorimotor neuropathy and alcoholism.[5]

Conservative measures to treat a CN event begin with offloading—whether with a cast, Charcot restraint orthotic walker (CROW), brace, and, in the case of skin breakdown, total contact casts.[10,11] When a patient presents with a CN that has progressed to a rigid deformity and/or with a wound resistant to healing, additional steps may be

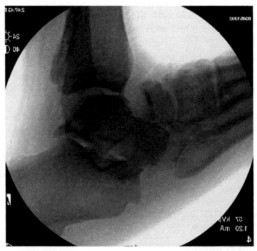

Fig. 2. Radiograph of a diabetic patient who experienced a proximal midfoot fracture dislocation with Charcot arthropathy.

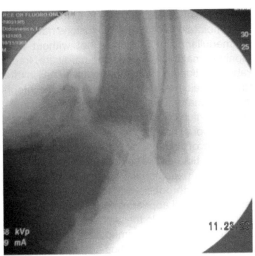

Fig. 3. Radiograph of a diabetic patient who experienced an ankle fracture dislocation with Charcot arthropathy.

warranted. With a rigid deformity and chronic wound, a patient is at great risk for infection and amputation as well as reduced quality of life.[7,12]

The goal of reconstruction in a patient with an ankle joint affected by CN is to restore alignment and stability to the ankle and hindfoot in an effort to provide a functional limb. The senior author's staged algorithm for the management of these patients begins with addressing the patient's medical status and ensuring a multispecialty approach (medicine, vascular surgery, infectious disease, physical therapy social work, and so on) before pursuing definitive surgical reconstruction.[10]

When nonoperative care has failed and the patient presents with wounds, infections, and instability, surgical intervention is warranted. Studies have demonstrated compromised successes and increased complications in CN reconstruction alongside patient comorbidities.[2,9] McCann and colleagues[9] noted in 151 cases that those who underwent ankle or subtalar reconstruction were 70% less likely to return to walking than those undergoing medial column reconstruction. These patients were also 3.3 times more likely to require amputation within 3 years after surgery. Rehabilitation following either a below-knee amputation or CN reconstruction is not a small task. The ultimate decision of whether to pursue surgical intervention for reconstruction versus a below-knee amputation is up to the patient with expert input from the surgeon.

Unlike healthy bone, the bone in the patient with CN is often diseased and noted to be weak, osteoporotic, and fragmented. Bone may exhibit decreased density as well as an overabundance of osteoclasts.[5,13] The role of treating bone affected by the disease pharmacologically is still unclear.[14,15] Well-accepted and traditional methods of internal fixation, including lag screws with plates, are usually insufficient to meet the demands of stabilizing bone commonly exhibited by CN. Surgical reconstruction in CN is commonly staged in the presence of infection and may include a combination of internal fixation, external fixation, and/or hybrid constructs.

Plate Fixation in Ankle Charcot

Given the severe deformities and the altered bone biology seen in CN, traditional constructs used for fusions such as screws alone in most scenarios should be replaced or supplemented by stronger, more rigid constructs.[16,17]

When addressing ankle joint destruction due to CN, intramedullary nail fixations for tibiocalcaneal (TC) and tibiotalocalcaneal (TTC) fusions have proved to be successful constructs.[18,19] Intramedullary nail fixation is not without potential complications including malpositioning, malunion, nonunion, hardware fracture, implant failure, and fracture. Desirable positioning of an intramedullary nail is often difficult especially the entrance point into the calcaneus. In addition to this, the integrity of the soft tissues and the ability to establish anatomic alignment must be taken into consideration by the surgeon. The calcaneus, which characteristically has a thin outer bony cortex and an abundance of cancellous bone, has weaker holding ability, therefore precise entrance is paramount for this type of fixation. In patients with nonpathologic anatomy, the calcaneus lies lateral to the tibia. In the senior author's experience, in seeing and performing revision surgeries in patients who have experienced ankle and hindfoot CN and a previously attempted arthrodesis with intramedullary nail fixation, he has often found that the intramedullary nail appears in good position on the lateral radiographs many times misleading the surgeon. In these cases, he has frequently identified failure in the appropriate placement of the intramedullary nail. Routinely the nail has been inserted more medially on the calcaneus thus not purchasing the body of the calcaneus leading to failure. In the senior author's experience the vast majority of failures of intramedullary nails occur in the calcaneus (**Figs. 4** and **5**).

The difficulty of precise placement and other postoperative complications associated with intramedullary nail fixation for TTC and TC fusions have encouraged the use of locking plate constructs for the rearfoot and ankle.[20–22] A cadaveric study by O'Neill and colleagues in 2008 demonstrated that screw fixation augmented with a lateral locking plate versus augmentation with an intramedullary nail may provide similar rigidity required for a TTC fusion.[23]

Early studies showcase the use of blade plates for the surgical treatment of tibiotalar (TC) or TTC fusions, which were originally designed for use in subtrochanteric femur fractures.[24] In addition, surgeons have used locking plates created for humeral and femoral fractures.[22] Modern technology now includes anatomic plates specifically for rearfoot and ankle fusions (**Figs. 6** and **7**).

A condylar blade plate with a fixed 90° to 95° angle has been used in TC or TTC arthrodesis. Originally described by Alvarez and colleagues[23] in 1994, it is placed laterally and tamped into the calcaneus just beneath the angle of Gissane (see Surgical Techniques section). In a biomechanical cadaver study, this construct was found to

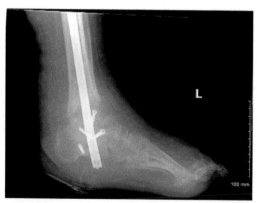

Fig. 4. Radiograph of a diabetic patient who underwent an attempt of a tibiotalocalcaneal arthrodesis with an intramedullary nail. The nail failed within the calcaneus.

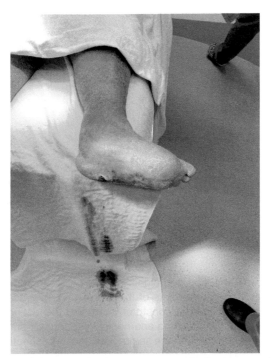

Fig. 5. Preoperative surgical view of a diabetic patient who had previously had an attempted tibiotalocalcaneal arthrodesis with an intramedullary nail that failed. The nail is now protruding through the calcaneus and is resulting in an infection.

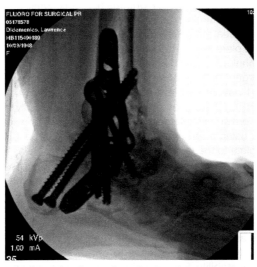

Fig. 6. An intraoperative lateral radiograph projection demonstrating a diabetic who had a tibiotalocalcaneal arthrodesis performed using a lateral-based plate along with fully threaded large cancellous screws. Note the multiple holes of fixation within the calcaneus, the talus, and the tibia.

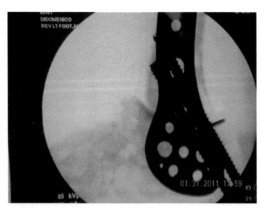

Fig. 7. An intraoperative lateral radiograph projection demonstrating an femoral locking plate prepared for fixation. Note the multiple holes of potential fixation in the "weaker" cancellous calcaneal bone.

have lower plastic deformation and higher stiffness than an intramedullary rod.[24] In addition, the plate offers more points of fixation distally. The use of a locking plate construct provides a rigid, stable construct while also respecting the biological demands of bone healing. With locking and nonlocking screws, surgeons can achieve compression and stability through the same plate. In a retrospective review of 30 patients (26 of whom had CN), fusion occurred in 28 patients by an average of 16 weeks. Of note, patients were non-weight-bearing for 3 months in a below-knee cast and progressed to weight-bearing the following 3 months[25] (**Fig. 8**).

Early on, proximal humeral locking plates provided a potential upgrade for the TC or TCC fusion construct. In 2007, Ahmad and colleagues reported successful union in 17 of 18 patients using the Proximal Humerus Internal Locking System (PHILOS) by Synthes, Paoli, Pa.[26] A cadaver study by Chodos and colleagues[27] compared a laterally based blade plate to a laterally placed proximal humeral locking plate. The investigators reported higher initial stiffness, torsional load to failure, and lower construct deformation than a blade plate for a TTC fusion construct; they also noted that placement of a blade plate is technically more difficult than that of locking plates and does not allow for screws in divergent orientations.[27] Another study by Shearman and colleagues[16] noted that 18 of 21 patients achieved fusion over an average 4.8 months (**Fig. 9**).

Like humeral locking plates, femoral locking plates, primarily intended for femoral condyle fractures, provide a suitable contour for TC and TTC fusions. In the senior author's experience, using a femoral locking plate for a TC or a TTC fusion provides a nicely contoured plate to the lateral tibia, calcaneus, and/or talus. One can place multiple locked or nonlocking bicortical screws into the calcaneus, which exhibits a thin cortex and an abundance of porous cancellous bone. The proximal holes in the plate allow for a combination of locking and/or nonlocking screws.[22]

Modern plating technology is specifically designed to contour ankle and rearfoot anatomy. It has been the senior author's experience to use 2 or 3 fully threaded large cancellous screws as positional screws. It is important to use the cortex-cortex technique allowing the fully threaded screws to act as positional screws and maintain length, strength, and stability. For example, a screw can be inserted from the posterior inferior cortex of the calcaneus into the distal anterior tibial cortex. In addition, these fully threaded cancellous screws provide fixation from a different anatomic location providing more stability. Also these fully threaded screws can be long and near the

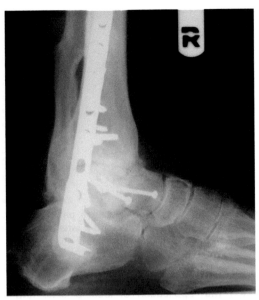

Fig. 8. Radiograph of a diabetic patient who suffers from diabetic peripheral neuropathy and a history of previous trauma and Charcot arthropathy. A previous attempt of a TTC arthrodesis failed. In this lateral radiograph a lateral-based blade plate was used in the surgical revision of the TTC arthrodesis.

length of an intramedullary nail. Based on what system the surgeon is choosing to use, the fully threaded screws can have a length of 100 to 150 mm. In addition, if the surgeon uses 2 or 3 fully threaded screws from cortex to cortex, the added diameter will often be equal to or larger than the diameter of the intramedullary nails on the market providing excellent stability. Arguably the multiple long fully threaded screws may provide more stiffness when compared with an intramedullary nail (**Fig. 10**).

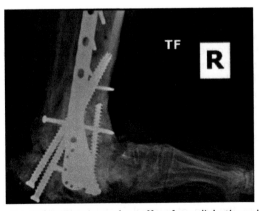

Fig. 9. Radiograph of a diabetic patient who suffers from diabetic peripheral neuropathy and a history of Charcot arthropathy and previous history of osteomyelitis. In this lateral radiograph a lateral-based humeral locking plate was used in the surgical reconstruction of a TTC arthrodesis.

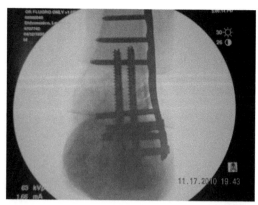

Fig. 10. An intraoperative anteroposterior view in a patient with Charcot arthropathy treated with 2 fully threaded cancellous screws and a lateral-based femoral locking plate. Note the multiple points of fixation in the calcaneus.

In cases in which there is compromise to the anterior or lateral soft tissue envelopes a posterior approach with application of locking plate and intramedullary fully threaded bicortical fixation can be used. The posterior approach to the ankle and/or subtalar joint provides a thick and well-vascularized soft tissue envelope and allows excellent exposure to the articular surfaces of the ankle and subtalar joints for TTC arthrodesis. Patzkowski and colleagues[28] found better visualization with a direct posterior approach with splitting of the Achilles tendon versus a posterior lateral approach based on anatomic structures observed. Didomenico and Sann[29] reported the successful posterior use of an anterior locking plate for an ankle and hindfoot arthrodesis. Hanson and colleagues[30] noted a 100% fusion rate in 10 patients with mild to moderate hindfoot and ankle deformity.[31] With the posterior approach awareness of anatomic structures is vital to reducing the risk of potential complications. Complications associated with this approach include injury to the sural nerve, flexor hallucis longus (FHL) tendons, as well as the anterior neurovascular structures during resection of the articular surfaces (**Fig. 11**).

Midfoot Charcot

In most patients who present with CN the isolated midfoot will be affected. In a systematic review of 1143 cases treated surgically, 59.5% of interventions were for midfoot Charcot arthropathy and 29.3% for ankle.[29,30] In surgical cases in which a patient presents with both ankle and hindfoot Charcot arthropathy, the surgeon needs to work from most straight/stable to less stable/less straight therefore surgically correcting the ankle before surgical repair of the midfoot. Once the ankle/hindfoot has been surgically addressed, the surgeon can better evaluate the midfoot and make appropriate surgical decisions. In cases involving both anatomic locations, the senior surgeon prefers to stage the surgeries because this can be a lot of physiologic stress on the patient and their respected limb. In addition, this can involve a lot of work and can be stressful for the surgeon as well.

Relative to surgical reconstructive efforts of the midfoot in cases with Charcot arthropathy, before the use of internal fixation, the surgical treatment generally included exostectomy, ulcer debridement and/or excision, realignment osteotomies, and possibly amputation.[29,32,33] As discussed earlier, the senior author prefers a staged approach if there is an ankle deformity that needs to be surgically addressed

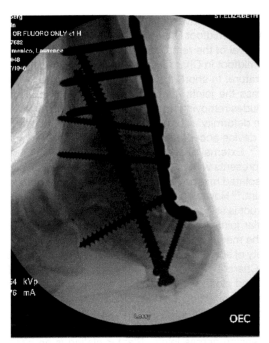

Fig. 11. Radiograph of a diabetic patient who has a history of Chariot arthropathy, positional arthrodesis failure, and a previous history of osteomyelitis. Because of the patient's previous history, a posterior approach was performed because of the healthy soft tissue envelope.

in combination with a midfoot deformity. In cases in which there is an ankle Charcot arthropathy involved, once osseous alignment and stability is achieved, the midfoot can be addressed in the same setting or as a staged approach.

In many situations, the CN progression has presented with a broken down foot, ulceration, and often osteomyelitis. The ulcer, infection, and/or osteomyelitis are secondary to the malaligned broken down foot. In scenarios with an infection or contamination, a combination of staged planned reconstruction is necessary. The initial stage consists of lengthening the posterior muscle group with an Achilles tendon lengthening or a gastrocnemius recession based on a Silfverskiöld examination.[33–35] Next, an incision, drainage, debridement of bone, and surgical debridement of the wound along with the bone is performed. Skin graft substitutes can be used in cases in which there is not an acutely infected surgical site. Once the bone debridement is performed (whether a rigid deformity or nonrigid), the surgeon needs to debride, resect diseased bone, and allow the deformity to become reducible. Once the deformity is reducible, it can be realigned using an external fixator, which can provide anatomic alignment and stability; this will also accomplish the offloading of the affected pathologic site. Typically negative pressure therapy is used to assist with wound management and closure. An infectious disease and vascular consults are commonly requested.

Once the wound is closed and the serum markers such as the white blood cell count, erythrocyte sedimentation rate, and C-reactive protein level are normal, the second portion of the planned, staged reconstruction is completed. At the time of the second staged reconstruction the external fixator is removed. This surgical reconstruction consists of additional bone resection removing any remaining diseased

Charcot/chronically infected/avascular bone[10] to the remaining healthy bleeding better-quality bone. For midfoot Charcot, this may include what is termed an "internal amputation," or removal of the remaining bone in the midfoot.

Addressing the midfoot in Charcot with a "superconstruct" approach is well documented in the literature. In short, the "superconstruct" means using plate, beam, or bolt fixation to cross the joints affected and include joints unaffected by CN. This approach also includes removing nonviable tissue or bone to shorten the foot to allow for reduction of the deformity without compromising other soft tissues and placing the strongest internal device accepted by the soft tissues in a biomechanically advantageous position.[36,37] External fixation may also be used as adjunct fixation. Midfoot Charcot primarily presents with disruption to the naviculocuneiform joints or tarsometatarsal joints. In isolated midfoot Charcot, addressing the equinus due to the Achilles tendon is paramount.[38] However, performing a subtalar joint fusion as well to "protect" the midfoot construct is still debated depending on the construct. A recent study suggested that subtalar joint fusion was associated with 80% lower complication rate than beaming of the medial column alone.[39]

Although a variety of screw, beam, and bolt constructs are possible, use of plate fixation in midfoot Charcot may provide a stronger construct offering stability and compression. Isolated plating of the midfoot begins with medial column stabilization or with intramedullary beaming or bolts. Plate application can be applied dorsal, medial (or dorsomedial), or plantar.[40,41] Dorsal plating is not recommended because it is weaker than screw fixation alone. Plantar plating is the most biomechanically sound given the tension across joints. Plantar plating is an effective fixation option for sagittal plane correction in the rocker-bottom deformity, especially at Lisfranc joint. However, placing a plantar plate presents a challenge to the surgeon in terms of dissection and placement of a contoured plate.[41] Simons and colleagues[42] showed no statistical difference between dorsal medial versus plantar plating with regard to stiffness and cycles to failure. Their constructs encompassed the navicular to the first metatarsal[42] (**Fig. 12**).

Surgical Techniques

In the author's experience, surgical reconstruction of an ankle and foot affected by CN that presents with an open wound and/or infection should be treated in a staged fashion. When the patient presents with an open wound and/or infection the first stage generally focuses on infection control, aggressive resection of the diseased or infected bone, specific identification of the pathogen, followed by reduction of the deformity, and wound care. The unstable deformity is reduced, put into anatomic alignment,

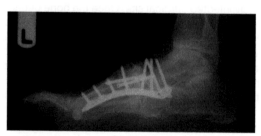

Fig. 12. A postoperative lateral radiograph demonstrating a plantar plate applied to the tension side of the Lisfranc and midfoot deformity. Note the positional screws inserted outside of the plate extending to the lateral aspect of the foot.

and stability is maintained with the use of a pin-to-bar external static multilevel external fixator until the reconstructive procedure.

If reconstruction of the ankle is necessary, this is the first level of deformity addressed once the external fixator is removed. The Silfverskiöld test is carried out to determine whether gastrocnemius or gastrosoleal equinus is present. If a gastrosoleal equinus is present a tendo-Achilles lengthening is performed using the traditional percutaneous hemisection approach.[33] If an isolated gastrocnemius recession is present, then it is preferred to perform an endoscopic gastric recession, and if an endoscopic recession cannot be obtained successfully then an open gastrocnemius recession can be performed.[33]

Plating for Tibiotalocalcaneal or Tibiocalcaneal Arthrodesis

A transfibular approach is used to access the TTC or TC joints. A full-thickness incision is made directly over the fibula. A fibular osteotomy is made about 10 to 15 cm proximal to the distal tip of the lateral malleolus. The syndesmosis is taken down using an osteotome and mallet. The distal portion of the fibula is removed. The most distal 2 cm of the fibula is split and used as a cortical cancellous autograft and used as an inlay graft or onlay graft. Another option is to decorticate the medial aspect of the fibular strut and use this as an inlay graft and as a biological plate.[43] Another option is to use the fibula as an intramedullary nail. In most cases the senior author splits the distal 2 cm and uses this as a cortical cancellous inlay graft to maintain length and anatomic position. The proximal portion of the fibular is put through a bone mill to aid in fusion and is mixed with the patient's blood. At the time of anesthesia, once the patient is induced, the anesthesia team harvests approximately 15 to 20 mL of the patient's blood and the author soaks the fibula grafts in this blood.

Most of the surgical procedure time is spent preparing the joint for fusion. Joint preparation is achieved with rongeurs, curettes, drills, osteotomes, mallets, and a high-speed bur. Again this is critical to resect all diseased, avascular, and necrotic bone along with any invaginated fibrous tissue.

The deformity is then reduced and temporarily fixated with large K-wire fixation. Next, 2 or 3 large fully threaded cancellous screws are placed from the posterior-inferior aspect of the calcaneus to superior-anterior obliquely across the subtalar and ankle and joints. If a third large cancellous screw is used, it is inserted from the anterior/inferior plantar cortex of the calcaneus to the posterior inferior tibia cortex. As previously mentioned, the diameter of a combination of 2 or 3 large fully threaded cancellous screws will typically result in a greater diameter than the largest nail on the market while providing bicortical purchase and maintaining length and position. Next the autogenous bone graft and if needed allograft cancellous bone chips are packed very tightly to the bony deficit. A lateral-based plate is applied to the lateral aspect of the calcaneus, talus (if present) and tibia; this is applied with a combination of locking and nonlocking screws. Nonlocking screws are used first to compress the plate to the bone and then locking the plate in place once anatomically positioned. The senior author's most sturdiest fixation construct includes utilization of a femoral locking plate placed laterally (**Figs. 13–15**).

In cases in which a posterior approach must be used a direct posterior incision is made overlying the Achilles tendon. During TTC arthrodesis the Achilles tendon can be released from its insertion and resected; this will provide excellent visualization and will provide good vascularity during healing because the avascular tendon is now absent. It will also allow for easier closure because there is less strain on the soft tissue envelope. The deep fascia is then incised and the FHL tendon with its muscle belly can now be visualized. The FHL is then retracted and dissection is carried

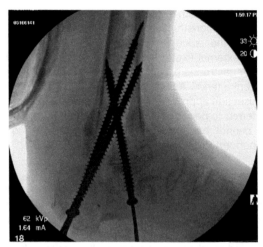

Fig. 13. An intraoperative lateral radiograph demonstrating 3 large cancellous screws inserted from the inferior calcaneal cortex to tibial cortex as positional screws. Note that there is no compression over the bone graft.

down to the posterior tibia, talus, and calcaneus. The articular surface of each joint is removed to healthy bleeding bone. Any deformity that is present is reduced and held in anatomic position with temporary pins and guidewires. Full threaded cancellous screws are then placed into the desired position. A locking plate is then fixated to

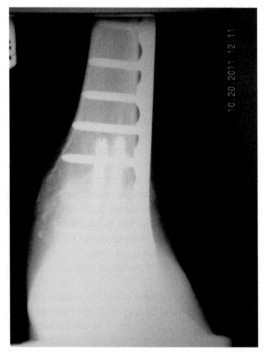

Fig. 14. A postoperative anteroposterior radiograph demonstrating good anatomic alignment with excellent fixation following a tibiotalocalcaneal arthrodesis using a femoral locking plate and fully threaded bicortical large cancellous screws.

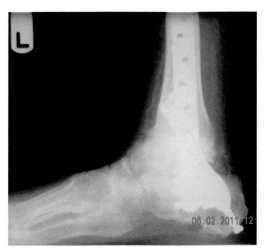

Fig. 15. A postoperative lateral radiograph demonstrating good anatomic alignment with excellent fixation following a tibiotalocalcaneal arthrodesis using a femoral locking plate and fully threaded bicortical large cancellous screws.

the tibia, talus, and calcaneus using a combination of locking and nonlocking screws.[29] The FHL muscle belly is incorporated in the closure of the deep soft tissue, which provides excellent coverage of the internal fixation.

When appropriately determined, a drain is used and then the deep tissues are closed using 0-vicryl and skin closed using 2-0 nylon sutures. The surgical wounds are dressed with betadine-soaked Adaptic, 4 × 4s gauze, and kling in a sterile compressive fashion. A univalve below-knee cast with a medial and lateral splint as well as a posterior splint is applied[44] (**Figs. 16** and **17**).

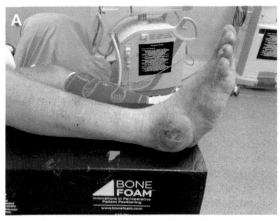
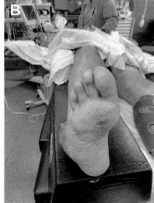

Fig. 16. (*A, B*) Preoperative clinical view of a patient who suffered from Charcot arthropathy with a large hindfoot and ankle varus deformity as well as a large bony mass causing a recurrent chronic ulceration leading to soft tissue envelope pathology; this was a staged planned reconstruction surgery. The initial surgery was to remove the large bony mass with culture and biopsy.

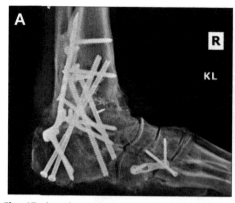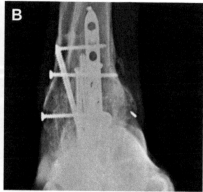

Fig. 17. (*A, B*) Postoperative anteroposterior and lateral radiographic views of a patient who suffered from Charcot arthropathy with a large hindfoot and ankle varus deformity as well as a large bony mass causing a recurrent chronic ulceration leading to soft tissue envelope pathology. Once the mass was removed and noted to be benign, a staged planned reconstruction surgery was performed consisting of correction of the tight posterior muscle group and a posterior approach performing TTC arthrodesis through the posterior corridor of the hindfoot and ankle.

Plating for Midfoot Arthrodesis

A medial incision is made overlying the midfoot and deepened down to bone maintaining full-thickness tissue layers. A multiplanar bone resection is performed to correct the underlying malalignment. Common malalignments are abducted, rotated into varus, and dorsiflexion. Typically this bony resection consists of a bone resection with the base being plantar and medial and the apex being lateral and dorsal in most cases; this allows the typical malaligned foot to be adducted, plantar flexed, and rotated into an anatomic neutral position. In scenarios in which the deformity is different, then the appropriate debridement of diseased bone needs to be resected to reduce the malalignment into anatomic alignment. Bone resection consists of diseased midfoot bone excised while also correcting the present deformity. Care is taken not to overadduct the foot and create a metatarsal adducts deformity or a "C"-shaped foot (this can become pathologic). The position is then held with large K-wires temporary fixation. Next, intramedullary screw fixation can be achieved creating good bone-to-bone contact at the plantar surfaces and then a medial base or plantar plate is applied for additional structural support. The other option is to use a plate (preferably a recon plate plantarly or a medial-based plate) using an eccentric loading technique with the plate obtaining compression.[41] Once this is achieved, structural positional screws are inserted outside and around the plate followed by bone grafting of the dorsal bony gaps. When applying the midfoot reconstruction plate it is applied with a combination of locking and nonlocking screws.

In cases in which there is both a rearfoot and midfoot deformity it is the authors' preference to perform a percutaneous calcaneal osteotomy using a Gigli saw.[33] When the talonavicular joint is involved, a 6.5 bolt is placed from the posterior lateral talus down the medial column to the proximal aspect of the first metatarsal (**Figs. 18–20**).

Postoperative Care

Postoperatively, the patient is placed in a univalve plaster cast and is non-weight-bearing.[44] This cast is kept intact for 2 weeks following surgery unless the provider

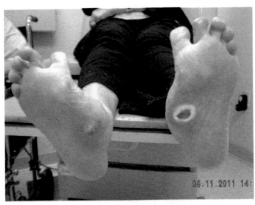

Fig. 18. Preoperative clinical view of a patient who suffered from bilateral Charcot arthropathy and diabetic foot ulcers.

is concerned for a wound complication, deep vein thrombosis, infection, and so on. A fiberglass below the knee cast is then applied for approximately 6 to 8 weeks and based on postoperative radiographs and soft tissue envelope. Following clinical and radiographic consolidation is confirmed via radiographs/and or computed tomographic scan, the transition to a customized CROW boot is facilitated and used for approximately 6 months. Following 6 months of successful use of a CROW walker, the senior author transitions the patients into an ankle-foot orthosis (AFO). The AFO is used for approximately 6 months and then converted to regular shoes or custom-made shoes if needed. If a TTC or a TC arthrodesis was performed, a rocker bottom will be used with the shoes to aid in ambulation. If there are concerns of a delay in the bony union, extended use of below-the-knee casting, contolled ankle motion (CAM) boot, CROW boot, or AFO are indicated and periodically evaluated with CT scans and serial radiographs.

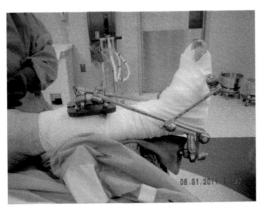

Fig. 19. Intraoperative clinical view of a patient who suffered from Charcot arthropathy, an equinus contracture, a diabetic foot ulcer, and osteomyelitis. A bone debridement and posterior muscle lengthening was performed with application of multilevel external fixator. Anatomic alignment was maintained along with a reduction of the deformity. The patient received intravenous antibiotics with the infectious disease team.

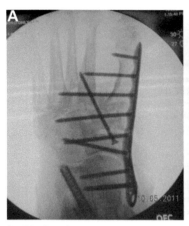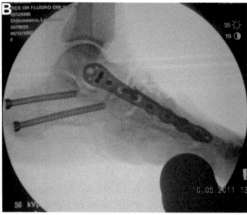

Fig. 20. (*A, B*) An intraoperative lateral radiograph demonstrating anatomic alignment an preparation for arthrodesis. A percutaneous calcaneal osteotomy was performed in combination with the midfoot and Lisfranc arthrodesis.

SUMMARY

Plate fixation for reduction and correction of ankle and midfoot CN includes a variety of approaches. The senior author's utilization of plating and treating an ankle and midfoot CN focuses on a staged approach. This approach includes addressing the wound, and infection, and osteomyelitis if present with wide aggressive soft tissue and bone resection before definitive internal fixation, resulting in surgical cure. For the ankle and hindfoot, a lateral approach is generally performed using a rigid construct such as a femoral locking plate. For the midfoot, a plantarly or medially placed plate construct is often performed. Both constructs are supplemented with screws outside of the plate fixation.

Ultimately, the surgeon's approach should address the underlying pathology so the surgeon can fundamentally correct the unbalanced pathologic foot and place it into an anatomic balanced aligned position in efforts of preventing reoccurrence. It is important to use a multidisciplinary approach to ensure the best patient outcome. If this approach presents difficulty or fails, the patient will be facing a significant revisional effort and or possible below-knee amputation.

CLINICS CARE POINTS

- Bone resection and removal of all diseased bone
- Reduction of the deformity to anatomic alignment
- Excellent rigid internal fixation is necessary for successful outcome
- The surgeon must have skills with internal fixation, external fixation, a good understanding of lower extremity vascular disease, and a good understanding of infectious disease and plastic surgical techniques of the lower extremity.

DISCLOSER

Relative to this article, there are no disclosures.

REFERENCES

1. Rosenbaum AJ, DiPreta JA. Classifications in brief: Eichenholtz classification of Charcot arthropathy. Clin Orthop Relat Res 2015;473(3):1168–71.
2. Shibata T, Tada K, Hashizume C. The results of arthrodesis of the ankle for leprotic neuroarthropathy. J Bone Joint Surg Am 1990;72:749–56.
3. Pinzur MS. Current concepts review: charcot arthropathy of the foot and ankle. Foot Ankle Int 2007;28(8):952–9.
4. Sanders LJ. The charcot foot: historical perspective 1827-2003. Diabetes Metab Res Rev 2004;20(Suppl 1):S4–8.
5. Frykberg RG, Belczyk R. Epidemiology of the charcot foot. Clin Podiatr Med Surg 2008;25(1):17–v.
6. Sinha S, Munichoodappa CS, Kozak GP. Neuro-arthropathy (Charcot joints) in diabetes mellitus: clinical study of 101 cases. Medicine 1972;51(3):191–210.
7. Sohn MW, Lee TA, Stuck RM, et al. Mortality risk of Charcot arthropathy compared with that of diabetic foot ulcer and diabetes alone. Diabetes Care 2009;32(5):816–21.
8. Rettedal D, Parker A, Popchak A, et al. Prognostic scoring system for patients undergoing reconstructive foot and ankle surgery for charcot neuroarthropathy: the charcot reconstruction preoperative prognostic score. J Foot Ankle Surg 2018;57(3):451–5.
9. McCann L, Zhu S, Pollard JD, et al. Success and survivorship following charcot reconstruction: a review of 151 cases. J Foot Ankle Surg 2021;60(3):535–40.
10. DiDomenico L, Flynn Z, Reed M. Treating charcot arthropathy is a challenge: explaining why my treatment algorithm has changed. Clin Podiatr Med Surg 2018;35(1):105–21.
11. Alvarez RG, Marini A, Schmitt C, et al. Stage I and II posterior tibial tendon dysfunction treated by a structured nonoperative management protocol: an orthosis and exercise program. Foot Ankle Int 2006;27(1):2–8.
12. Sochocki MP, Verity S, Atherton PJ, et al. Health related quality of life in patients with Charcot arthropathy of the foot and ankle. Foot Ankle Surg 2008;14(1):11–5.
13. Baumhauer JF, O'Keefe RJ, Schon LC, et al. Cytokine-induced osteoclastic bone resorption in charcot arthropathy: an immunohistochemical study. Foot Ankle Int 2006;27(10):797–800.
14. Jude EB, Selby PL, Burgess J, et al. Bisphosphonates in the treatment of Charcot neuroarthropathy: a double-blind randomised controlled trial. Diabetologia 2001;44(11):2032–7.
15. Petrova NL, Edmonds ME. Medical management of Charcot arthropathy. Diabetes Obes Metab 2013;15(3):193–7.
16. Shearman AD, Eleftheriou KI, Patel A, et al. Use of a proximal humeral locking plate for complex ankle and hindfoot fusion. J Foot Ankle Surg 2016;55(3):612–8.
17. Ögüt T, Yontar NS. Surgical treatment options for the diabetic charcot hindfoot and ankle deformity. Clin Podiatr Med Surg 2017;34(1):53–67.
18. Mendicino RW, Catanzariti AR, Saltrick KR, et al. Tibiotalocalcaneal arthrodesis with retrograde intramedullary nailing. J Foot Ankle Surg 2004;43(2):82–6.
19. Pelton K, Hofer JK, Thordarson DB. Tibiotalocalcaneal arthrodesis using a dynamically locked retrograde intramedullary nail. Foot Ankle Int 2006;27(10):759–63.
20. Thordarson DB, Chang D. Stress fractures and tibial cortical hypertrophy after tibiotalocalcaneal arthrodesis with an intramedullary nail. Foot Ankle Int 1999;20(8):497–500.

21. Jehan S, Shakeel M, Bing AJ, et al. The success of tibiotalocalcaneal arthrodesis with intramedullary nailing–a systematic review of the literature. Acta Orthop Belg 2011;77(5):644–51.

22. DiDomenico LA, Wargo-Dorsey M. Tibiotalocalcaneal arthrodesis using a femoral locking plate. J Foot Ankle Surg 2012;51(1):128–32.

23. O'Neill PJ, Logel KJ, Parks BG, et al. Rigidity comparison of locking plate and intramedullary fixation for tibiotalocalcaneal arthrodesis. Foot Ankle Int 2008;29(6): 581–6.

24. Chiodo CP, Acevedo JI, Sammarco VJ, et al. Intramedullary rod fixation compared with blade-plate-and-screw fixation for tibiotalocalcaneal arthrodesis: a biomechanical investigation. J Bone Joint Surg Am 2003;85(12):2425–8.

25. Myerson MS, Alvarez RG, Lam PW. Tibiocalcaneal arthrodesis for the management of severe ankle and hindfoot deformities. Foot Ankle Int 2000;21(8):643–50.

26. Ahmad J, Pour AE, Raikin SM. The modified use of a proximal humeral locking plate for tibiotalocalcaneal arthrodesis. Foot Ankle Int 2007;28(9):977–83.

27. Chodos MD, Parks BG, Schon LC, et al. Blade plate compared with locking plate for tibiotalocalcaneal arthrodesis: a cadaver study. Foot Ankle Int 2008;29(2): 219–24.

28. Patzkowski JC, Kirk KL, Orr JD, et al. Quantification of posterior ankle exposure through an achilles tendon-splitting versus posterolateral approach. Foot Ankle Int 2012;33(10):900–4.

29. Didomenico LA, Sann P. Posterior approach using anterior ankle arthrodesis locking plate for tibiotalocalcaneal arthrodesis. J Foot Ankle Surg 2011;50(5):626–9.

30. Hanson TW, Cracchiolo A. The use of a 95 blade plate and a posterior approach to achieve tibiotalocalcaneal arthrodesis. Foot Ankle Int 2002;23:704–10.

31. Hammit MD, Hobgood ER, Tarquinio TA. Midline posterior approach to the ankle and hindfoot. Foot Ankle Int 2006;27:711–5.

32. Nickisch F, Avilucea FR, Beals T, et al. Open posterior approach for tibiotalar arthrodesis. Foot Ankle Clin 2011;16(1):103–14.

33. DiDomenico LA, Adams HB, Garchar D. Endoscopic gastrocnemius recession for the treatment of gastrocnemius equinus. J Am Podiatr Med Assoc 2005; 95(4):410–3.

34. Saxena A, Gollwitzer H, Widtfeldt A, et al. Endoscopic gastrocnemius recession as therapy for gastrocnemius equinus. Z Orthop Unfall 2007;145(4):499–504.

35. Lowery NJ, Woods JB, Armstrong DG, et al. Surgical management of Charcot neuroarthropathy of the foot and ankle: a systematic review. Foot Ankle Int 2012;33(2):113–21.

36. Sammarco VJ. Superconstructs in the treatment of charcot foot deformity: plantar plating, locked plating, and axial screw fixation. Foot Ankle Clin 2009;14(3): 393–407.

37. Alrashidi Y, Hügle T, Wiewiorski M, et al. Surgical treatment options for the diabetic charcot midfoot deformity. Clin Podiatr Med Surg 2017;34(1):43–51.

38. Kwaadu KY. Charcot reconstruction: understanding and treating the deformed charcot neuropathic arthropathic foot. Clin Podiatr Med Surg 2020;37(2):247–61.

39. Manchanda K, Wallace SB, Ahn J, et al. Charcot midfoot reconstruction: does subtalar arthrodesis or medial column fixation improve outcomes? J Foot Ankle Surg 2020;59(6):1219–23.

40. Tan EW, Schon LC. plate fixation techniques for midfoot and forefoot charcot arthropathy. The surgical management of the diabetic foot and ankle. Springer International Publishing; 2016. p. 117–31.

41. Garchar D, DiDomenico LA, Klaue K. Reconstruction of Lisfranc joint dislocations secondary to Charcot neuroarthropathy using a plantar plate. J Foot Ankle Surg 2013;52(3):295–7.

42. Simons P, Sommerer T, Zderic I, et al. Biomechanical investigation of two plating systems for medial column fusion in foot. PLoS One 2017;12(2):e0172563.

43. Ley D, et al. "Can biological fibular plates provide viable fixation for tibiocalcaneal arthrodesis?" Hmpgloballearningnetwork.com, Podiatry Today. 2020. Available at: https://www.hmpgloballearningnetwork.com/site/podiatry/can-biological-fibular-plates-provide-viable-fixation-tibiocalcaneal-arthrodesis. Accessed April 8, 2020.

44. DiDomenico LA, Sann P. Univalve split plaster cast for postoperative immobilization in foot and ankle surgery. J Foot Ankle Surg 2013;52(2):260–2.

Nerve Decompression and Distal Transtibial Amputation

Edgardo R. Rodriguez- Collazo, DPM[a],
Stephanie Oexeman, DPM, AACFAS, DABPM[b],
Lauren L. Schnack, DPM, MS, AACFAS, FACPM[c,*]

KEYWORDS

- Transtibial amputation • Neuropathy • Entrapment • Nutrition

KEY POINTS

- Before surgical intervention, the patient must be evaluated by a neurophysiologist along the course of the entire affected nerve.
- At least 2 successful proximal nerve blocks need to be conducted before determining appropriate surgical intervention.
- The distal transtibial amputation has the option to use a bone bridge in order to stabilize the tibia-fibula syndesmosis for weight bearing.

INTRODUCTION ON NERVE DECOMPRESSION

Approximately 20% of patients with diabetic peripheral neuropathy (DPN) endorse painful sensations such as prickling, stabbing, and burning pain that reflect small-fiber involvement. Although glycemic control is crucial to delay the onset and progression of DPN, there have been many reports on the use of decompression nerve surgery to aid in the treatment of DPN.[1]

Double crush syndrome can occur in patients with a proximal and/or distal entrapment site of a nerve along with systemic factors such as diabetes, causing increased sorbitol within the neural structures.[2,3] In 2007, Dellon reported reduced pain, reduced reulceration rate, and improved sensation in most of the patients with DPN who underwent decompression of lower limb nerves.[1,4] Although the data on decompressive nerve surgery for DPN in the literature are inconclusive, there are proponents who

[a] Department of Surgery, Ascension Saint Joseph - Chicago, Laboure Outpatient Clinic, 2913 North Commonwealth Avenue, Chicago, IL 60657, USA; [b] Department of Surgery, Oexeman Foot and Ankle, PLLC, Ascension Saint Joseph - Chicago, 2913 North Commonwealth Avenue, Suite 425, Chicago, IL 60657, USA; [c] Ascension Saint Joseph - Chicago, Podiatric Fellow Office Suite 425, 2913 North Commonwealth Avenue, Chicago, IL 60657, USA
* Corresponding author.
E-mail address: laurenlschnackdpmms@gmail.com

Clin Podiatr Med Surg 39 (2022) 695–704
https://doi.org/10.1016/j.cpm.2022.05.009
0891-8422/22/© 2022 Elsevier Inc. All rights reserved.

view the surgery as a promising therapy for the properly selected patients with DPN, noting that unproven is not equivalent to unnecessary and unnecessary does not equate to ineffective or harmful.[1,4,5]

Diabetic patients with external entrapment of lower limb peripheral nerves can potentially benefit from surgical decompression of the external compression site. A meta-analysis of clinical studies that have performed decompression of the tibial nerve branches at the level of the ankle in DPN reported relief in 80% of the patients from a mean of 8.5 on the VAS to 2.0 and demonstrated 80% of the patients recover more than just protective sensation.[4]

Peripheral nerve decompression is performed in the patient with a neuropathy who has an external compression of a peripheral nerve in a known site of anatomic narrowing.[1,4,6] Decompression can be performed in all or one of the following nerves: common peroneal nerve at the level of the fibular neck, deep peroneal nerve, superficial peroneal nerve, and the tibial nerve and its branches. Electrodiagnostic and clinic examination findings should aid in the surgeon's choice in performing decompressions. Dellon reports that the presence of a positive Hoffmann-Tinel sign over the tibial nerve in the tarsal tunnel gives a 92% positive predictive value for good to excellent results after nerve decompression in the diabetic with neuropathy and 88% in the patient with idiopathic neuropathy.[6] The investigators suggest performing ultrasound-guided nerve blocks proximal to the point of maximal tenderness, or Hoffmann-Tinel location, with 2 cc of the local anesthetic of the physician's choice. If the patient obtains pain relief after the nerve blocks, this suggests that the patient may respond well to surgical intervention and that the appropriate location of the nerve pathology was identified.[7]

Patients should be referred to a neurophysiologist when there is a suspected peripheral nerve injury. Electromyography and nerve conduction studies will determine which neural structures are affected, such as the myelin and axons. The results of the nerve conduction studies determine which neural structures are disrupted. The slowing of the latencies demonstrates disruption of the myelin and decreased amplitudes demonstrates axonal disruption.[7]

If DPN decompression surgery is to be performed, it should be addressed in a reconstructable zone of injury. If the skin is atrophic, indurated, or with poor vascularity, the surgical intervention is to be performed in a reconstructable zone with healthy tissue and vascularized wound bed. Orthoplastic approaches respect the soft tissue integrity, and incisions are made in regard to lower limb perforators and vascular structures.[7]

INTRODUCTION ON DISTAL TRANSTIBIAL AMPUTATION

It has been reported that 30% to 50% of patients who have undergone major lower limb amputations experience chronic pain of varying causes with the most commonly reported causes either being neuroma pain or phantom limb pain and often interferes with wearing a prosthetic. This constant pain has shown to decrease quality of life while increasing the risk of depression and having a negative impact on patients' relationships.[8]

The distal transtibial amputation discussed in this article offers an osteomyoplastic approach with active neural reconstruction compared with the traditional below-knee amputation and traction neurectomies commonly performed. With the distal transtibial amputation, after the surgical tibial resection, 10 to 15 cm of the tibia must remain in order to have an adequate prosthetic fit. The distal end of the stump and the weight-bearing surface should be at least 17 cm in order to obtain an integrated foot and pylon shock-absorbing system.[9] The Ertl technique incorporates the bone bridge to provide a stable weight-bearing surface for a prosthetic.[9]

To help reduce, or prevent, phantom limb pain, the distal transtibial amputation with active reconstructive nerve repairs is an osteomyoplastic approach to help prevent neuroma formation and phantom limb pain. The active, or reconstruction, options have been documented and consist of allograft or autograft reconstruction with conduit repair, end-to-side neurorrhaphy, targeted muscle reinnervation (TMR), regenerative peripheral nerve interface (RPNI), and vascularized peripheral nerve interface (VRPNI).[10]

Active Neural Reconstruction Options for Distal Transtibial Amputation

TMR is a reconstructive nerve option. Once transection of the nerve occurs, the nerve is coapted to a superficial motor nerve branch of a neighboring muscle. The native nerve will reinnervate that muscle; this is in order to prevent a painful neuroma formation.[11] TMR is still a relatively new surgery, and although recent literature reports are promising, further studies and investigations are needed.

An RPNI is after a neurectomy of the nerve; the nerve is enveloped within an elevated free tissue muscle graft. Over time there is neovascularization from the surrounding wound bed and neurotization of the elevated muscle graft.[12]

Patient Indications

Preoperatively, the patient must be evaluated in respect to vascular status and nutrition. To ensure adequate healing potential, the ankle-brachial index should be greater than 0.5, the transcutaneous oxygen level should be greater than 20 mm Hg, the serum albumin level should be greater than 2.5 g/dL, and the absolute lymphocyte count should be greater than 1500/uL.[13]

The vascular service should be consulted before determination of the amputation site. Modalities such as the handheld Doppler, infrared camera, and computed tomography angiography are critical tools used for preoperative surgical planning. Smartphone thermography, coupled with the use of the doppler, has also been introduced to determine location of perforators and potential viability. This modality can be used preoperatively, intraoperatively, and postoperatively to determine point-of-care progress.[14–16]

Surgical Procedure

The patient is placed in a supine position. Attention is directed to the distal aspect of the lower limb. The medial border of the tibia and anterior and posterior borders of the fibula are to be identified and marked. The anterior crest of the tibia should be marked approximately 10 cm proximal to the ankle joint in order to identify the location of the tibial cut. A fish-mouth incision is then drawn 3 to 4 cm distal to the location of the tibial cut to ensure adequate soft tissue coverage is available. The corners of this fish-mouth incision are located midline between the anterior and posterior borders of the fibula and approximately 1 cm posterior to the posteromedial border of the tibia to preserve the peroneal and posterior tibial perforators (**Figs. 1** and **2**). As much viable soft tissue as possible is preserved for the posterior flap. Utilization of a Doppler ultrasound and thermal imaging preoperatively can aid in surgical planning in order to avoid perforators where possible[16] (see **Figs. 1** and **2**).

The incision is made through the subcutaneous tissue. Starting medially, neurovascular structures are identified. Each nerve is isolated and tagged, whereas vascular structures are identified and ligated. Next, the incision is deepened to the tibial periosteum, and sharp dissection is used to expose the tibia and fibula. A retractor is

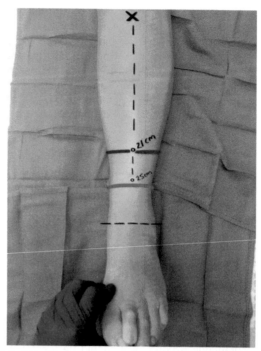

Fig. 1. A fish-mouth incision is mapped accordingly preoperatively. The tibial resection takes place approximately 10 cm proximal to the ankle joint. (*Photos courtesy of* Dr. Stephanie Oexeman, Chicago, IL.)

used and placed along the posterior aspect of the tibia and fibula to protect the posterior neurovascular bundle, and the tibial and fibular osteotomy is performed (**Fig. 3**). After the osteotomies are made, the foot is then able to be flexed at the amputation site, allowing the posterior flap to be completed (**Fig. 4**).

Next, a small portion of the fibula (which can be taken from the distal amputated specimen) is used as a bone bridge between the distal aspect of the fibula and tibia.

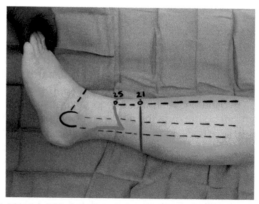

Fig. 2. A fish-mouth incision is mapped accordingly preoperatively. The tibial resection takes place approximately 10 cm proximal to the ankle joint. (*Photos courtesy of* Dr. Stephanie Oexeman, Chicago, IL.)

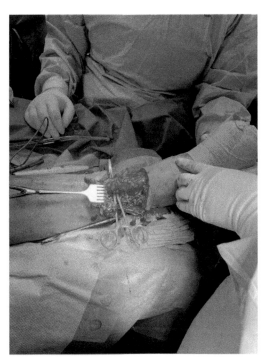

Fig. 3. A retractor is placed behind the posterior aspect of the tibia in preparation of the tibial osteotomy; this protects the posterior neurovascular package. (*Photo courtesy of* Dr. Edgardo Rodriguez-Collazo, Chicago, IL.)

The lateral tibial cortical bone and medial aspect of the fibula should be decorticalized to bleeding bone, and the portion of the fibula is then pressed fit between the fibula and tibia, which is fixated by surgeon's choice. The bridge between the tibia and fibula acts as a syndesmosis; this can consist of a fibula autograft, a 3.5-mm screw, Kirschner wire, or TightRope from Arthrex.[9] This procedure is performed with the goal of creating an osseous synostosis as originally described by Ertl in 1949.[9,17] The bone bridge osteoplastic component (**Fig. 5**) of this procedure adds surgical time intraoperatively, but this is indicated in motivated, active patients[9] (see **Fig. 5**).

Then, each nerve is isolated, a neurectomy of the nerve is performed to healthy bleeding tissue, and either a TMR or a regenerative peripheral nerve interface is performed to actively reconstruct the nerve ends in order to prevent painful neuroma formation. Depending on the soft tissue availability, it is the investigator's preference to perform a tibial nerve conduit—allograft assisted target muscle reinnervation to the soleus muscle when possible. Each reconstructed nerve is placed posterior to the tibia.

Transposition of the anterior, posterior, and lateral muscular group is performed at the distal tibia-fibula articulation. A drain should be placed for management of postoperative bleeding and hematoma formation, and the surgical site is closed per surgeon's choice. The surgical demonstration is depicted in **Figs. 1–5** and **Figs. 6–9**.

DISCUSSION

There are 2 million amputees in the United States with 25% of the amputees suffering from chronic phantom limb pain, which can make wearing a prosthesis painful and

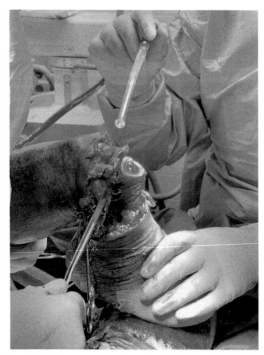

Fig. 4. After the tibia and fibula osteotomy is made, the foot can be flexed for easier access in completing the posterior flap. (*Photo courtesy of* Dr. Edgardo Rodriguez-Collazo, Chicago, IL.)

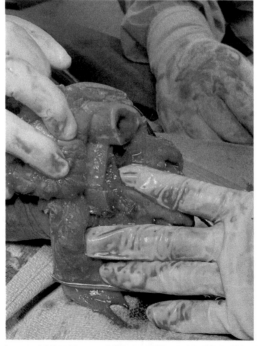

Fig. 5. Bone bridge between the tibia and fibula. (*Photo courtesy of* Dr. Edgardo Rodriguez-Collazo, Chicago, IL.)

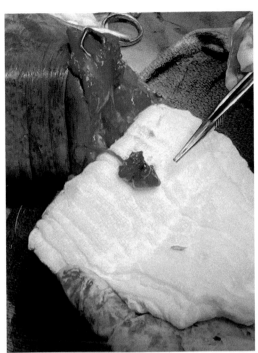

Fig. 6. Regenerative peripheral nerve interface of the saphenous nerve. (*Photo courtesy of* Dr. Edgardo Rodriguez-Collazo, Chicago, IL.)

result in a less active patient.[18] Revisional procedures such as TMR can be primary or secondary procedures for the treatment of phantom limb pain and neuromas.[8]

The distal transtibial osteomyoplastic amputation along with active reconstruction of neural structures can be used to provide a highly functional residual limb.[9]

A retrospective chart review of 294 amputations and 270 patients was conducted from 2004 to 2011, each of which underwent a transtibial amputation with a posterior myocutaneous flap involving a triceps surae myodesis. The purpose of this posterior myocutaneous flap is to provide adequate soft tissue coverage. Data were obtained from 192 patients after an average follow-up of 18.4 months. The cohort had a 75% ambulation rate, 12% stump wound incidence, 24% surgical revision rate, and 2% transfemoral amputation rate conversion. The investigators concluded the posterior myocutaneous flap is a reliable, stable, durable approach to soft tissue coverage in a transtibial amputation.[19]

Woo and colleagues reported on a series of patients who underwent RPNI for post-amputation neuroma pain. This study included 16 patients who collectively had 46 RPNIs performed. At 7.5-month follow-up, there was a 71% reduction in neuroma pain and 53% reduction in phantom limb pain. Out of 16 patients, 2 patients experienced neuroma pain, different from the surgical site.[8,12]

The TMR and RPNI aim to satisfy the nerve end and give the transected nerve a job to do.[10] TMR can be used in conjunction with a vascularized peripheral nerve interface as well.[20] A VRPNI is similar to an RPNI in that it is a denervated muscle cuff, but a pedicle is present so it remains vascularized. Valerio and colleagues discuss performing a TMR, and vascularized RPNI provides a denervated muscle cuff that is still vascularized, which can serve as a buffer for axonal escape through the TMR and can serve as an additional muscle target.[20]

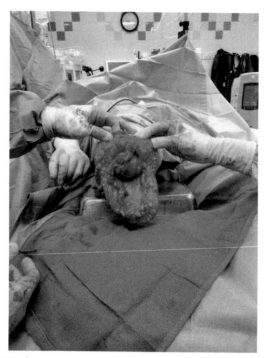

Fig. 7. Intraoperative photograph of the posterior muscle group over the distal aspect of the tibia and fibula. This takes place after each nerve is identified and reconstructed using targeted muscle reinnervation or regenerative peripheral nerve interface. These reconstructed nerves are placed posterior to the tibia and fibula. (*Photo courtesy of* Dr. Edgardo Rodriguez-Collazo, Chicago, IL.)

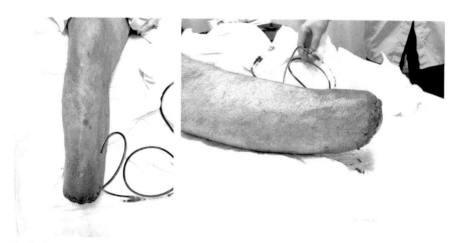

Fig. 8. Postoperative views of the reconstructive distal transtibial amputation. (*Photos courtesy of* Dr. Edgardo Rodriguez-Collazo, Chicago, IL.)

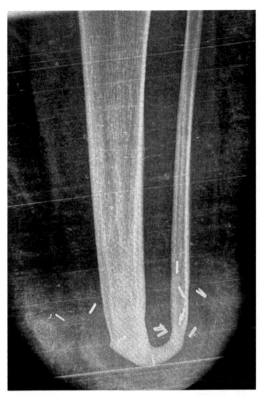

Fig. 9. Radiograph demonstrating distal transtibial amputation with consolidation of bone bridge between the tibia and fibula. (*Photo courtesy of* use by Dr. Edgardo Rodriguez-Collazo, Chicago, IL.)

TMR and RPNI are a reproducible procedure, which is reconstructive and restores physiologic continuity in order to prevent painful neuroma formation postoperatively.[18] Although these procedures provide promising early results in reducing neuroma pain and phantom limb pain, further long-term studies are needed.

CLINICS CARE POINTS

- The patient may have multifocal neuropathy due to multiple causes of nerve entrapment.
- Prior to distal transtibial amputation surgical intervention, the patient must be nutritionally optimized and evaluated with vascular testing.
- Active reconstruction peripheral nerve interventions are used in the osteomyoplastic distal transtibial amputation in order to prevent neuroma formation and phantom limb pain.

REFERENCES

1. Albers JW, Jacobson R. Decompression nerve surgery for diabetic neuropathy: a structured review of published clinical trials. Diabetes Metab Syndr Obes 2018; 11:493–514.

2. Cohen BH, Gaspar MP, Daniels AH, et al. Multifocal neuropathy: expanding the scope of double crush syndrome. J Hand Surg 2016;41(12):1171–5.
3. Kaur S, Pandhi P, Dutta P. Painful diabetic neuropathy: an update. Ann Neurosci 2011;18(4):168.
4. Dellon AL. Neurosurgical prevention of ulceration and amputation by decompression of lower extremity peripheral nerves in diabetic neuropathy: update 2006. Acta Neurochir Suppl 2007;100:149–51.
5. Nickerson DS. Comments on a proposal to limit Medicare coverage of nerve decompression surgery (electronic citation); 20181-4. Available at: www.dellon.com/8.pdf. Accessed October 1, 2021.
6. Lee C, Dellon AL. Prognostic ability of Tinel sign in determining outcome for decompression surgery decompression surgery in diabetic and non-diabetic neuropathy. Ann Plast Surg 2004;53:523–7.
7. Ward KL, Rodriguez-Collazo ER. Surgical treatment protocol for peripheral nerve dysfunction of the lower extremity: a systematic approach. Clin Podiatric Med Surg 2021;38(1):73–82.
8. Peters BR, Russo SA, West JM, et al. Targeted muscle reinnervation for the management of pain in the setting of major limb amputation. SAGE open Med 2020;8. 2050312120959180.
9. Taylor BC, Poka A. Osteomyoplastic transtibial amputation: the Ertl technique. J Am Acad Orthop Surg 2016;24(4):259–65.
10. Eberlin KR, Ducic I. Surgical algorithm for neuroma management: a changing treatment paradigm. Plast Reconstr Surg Glob Open 2018;6(10):e1952.
11. Valerio IL, Dumanian GA, Jordan SW, et al. Preemptive treatment of phantom and residual limb pain with targeted muscle reinnervation at the time of major limb amputation. J Am Coll Surg 2019;228(3):217–26.
12. Woo SL, Kung TA, Brown DL, et al. Regenerative peripheral nerve interfaces for the treatment of postamputation neuroma pain: a pilot study. Plast Reconstr Surg Glob Open 2016;4(12):e1038.
13. Pinzur MS, Stuck RM, Sage R, et al. Syme ankle disarticulation in patients with diabetes. J Bone Joint Surg Am 2003;85(9):1667–72.
14. Pereira N, Hallock GG. Smartphone thermography for lower extremity local flap perforator mapping. J Reconstr Microsurg 2021;37(01):059–66.
15. Pereira N, Valenzuela D, Mangelsdorff G, et al. Detection of perforators for free flap planning using smartphone thermal imaging: a concordance study with computed tomographic angiography in 120 perforators. Plast Reconstr Surg 2018;141(3):787–92.
16. Oexeman S, Ward KL. Understanding the arterial anatomy and dermal perfusion of the lower extremity with clinical application. Clin Podiatric Med Surg 2020; 37(4):743–9.
17. Ertl J. Uber amputationstumpfe. Chirurg 1949;20:218–24.
18. Bowen JB, Wee CE, Kalik J, et al. Targeted muscle reinnervation to improve pain, prosthetic tolerance, and bioprosthetic outcomes in the amputee. Adv Wound Care 2017;6(8):261–7.
19. Brown BJ, Iorio ML, Klement M, et al. Outcomes after 294 transtibial amputations with the posterior myocutaneous flap. Int J Low Extrem Wounds 2014;13(1): 33–40.
20. Valerio I, Schulz SA, West J, et al. Targeted muscle reinnervation combined with a vascularized pedicled regenerative peripheral nerve interface. Plast Reconstr Surg Glob Open 2020;8(3):e2689.

UNITED STATES POSTAL SERVICE®
Statement of Ownership, Management, and Circulation
(All Periodicals Publications Except Requester Publications)

1. Publication Title	2. Publication Number		3. Filing Date
CLINICS IN PODIATRIC MEDICINE & SURGERY	000 – 707		9/18/2022

4. Issue Frequency	5. Number of Issues Published Annually	6. Annual Subscription Price
JAN, APR, JUL, OCT	4	$319.00

7. Complete Mailing Address of Known Office of Publication (Not printer) (Street, city, county, state, and ZIP+4®)

ELSEVIER INC.
230 Park Avenue, Suite 800
New York, NY 10169

Contact Person
Malathi Samayan

Telephone (Include area code)
91-44-4299-4507

8. Complete Mailing Address of Headquarters or General Business Office of Publisher (Not printer)

ELSEVIER INC.
230 Park Avenue, Suite 800
New York, NY 10169

9. Full Names and Complete Mailing Addresses of Publisher, Editor, and Managing Editor (Do not leave blank)

Publisher (Name and complete mailing address)

DOLORES MELONI, ELSEVIER INC.
1600 JOHN F KENNEDY BLVD. SUITE 1800
PHILADELPHIA, PA 19103-2899

Editor (Name and complete mailing address)

MEGAN ASHDOWN, ELSEVIER INC.
1600 JOHN F KENNEDY BLVD. SUITE 1800
PHILADELPHIA, PA 19103-2899

Managing Editor (Name and complete mailing address)

PATRICK MANLEY, ELSEVIER INC.
1600 JOHN F KENNEDY BLVD. SUITE 1800
PHILADELPHIA, PA 19103-2899

10. Owner (Do not leave blank. If the publication is owned by a corporation, give the name and address of the corporation immediately followed by the names and addresses of all stockholders owning or holding 1 percent or more of the total amount of stock. If not owned by a corporation, give the names and addresses of the individual owners. If owned by a partnership or other unincorporated firm, give its name and address as well as those of each individual owner. If the publication is published by a nonprofit organization, give its name and address.)

Full Name	Complete Mailing Address
WHOLLY OWNED SUBSIDIARY OF REED/ELSEVIER, US HOLDINGS	1600 JOHN F KENNEDY BLVD. SUITE 1800 PHILADELPHIA, PA 19103-2899

11. Known Bondholders, Mortgagees, and Other Security Holders Owning or Holding 1 Percent or More of Total Amount of Bonds, Mortgages, or Other Securities. If none, check box. ▶ ☐ None

Full Name	Complete Mailing Address
N/A	

12. Tax Status (For completion by nonprofit organizations authorized to mail at nonprofit rates) (Check one)
The purpose, function, and nonprofit status of this organization and the exempt status for federal income tax purposes:
☒ Has Not Changed During Preceding 12 Months
☐ Has Changed During Preceding 12 Months (Publisher must submit explanation of change with this statement)

PS Form 3526, July 2014 [Page 1 of 4 (see instructions page 4)] PSN: 7530-01-000-9931   PRIVACY NOTICE: See our privacy policy on www.usps.com.

---

13. Publication Title			14. Issue Date for Circulation Data Below
CLINICS IN PODIATRIC MEDICINE & SURGERY			JULY 2022

15. Extent and Nature of Circulation			Average No. Copies Each Issue During Preceding 12 Months	No. Copies of Single Issue Published Nearest to Filing Date
a. Total Number of Copies (Net press run)			163	149
b. Paid Circulation (By Mail and Outside the Mail)	(1)	Mailed Outside-County Paid Subscriptions Stated on PS Form 3541 (include paid distribution above nominal rate, advertiser's proof copies, and exchange copies)	100	91
	(2)	Mailed In-County Paid Subscriptions Stated on PS Form 3541 (include paid distribution above nominal rate, advertiser's proof copies, and exchange copies)	0	0
	(3)	Paid Distribution Outside the Mails Including Sales Through Dealers and Carriers, Street Vendors, Counter Sales, and Other Paid Distribution Outside USPS®	13	11
	(4)	Paid Distribution by Other Classes of Mail Through the USPS (e.g., First-Class Mail®)	0	0
c. Total Paid Distribution (Sum of 15b (1), (2), (3), and (4))		▶	113	102
d. Free or Nominal Rate Distribution (By Mail and Outside the Mail)	(1)	Free or Nominal Rate Outside-County Copies included on PS Form 3541	34	31
	(2)	Free or Nominal Rate In-County Copies Included on PS Form 3541	0	0
	(3)	Free or Nominal Rate Copies Mailed at Other Classes Through the USPS (e.g., First-Class Mail)	0	0
	(4)	Free or Nominal Rate Distribution Outside the Mail (Carriers or other means)	0	0
e. Total Free or Nominal Rate Distribution (Sum of 15d (1), (2), (3) and (4))		▶	34	31
f. Total Distribution (Sum of 15c and 15e)		▶	147	133
g. Copies not Distributed (See Instructions to Publishers #4 (page #3))		▶	16	16
h. Total (Sum of 15f and g)		▶	163	149
i. Percent Paid (15c divided by 15f times 100)		▶	76.87%	76.69%

* If you are claiming electronic copies, go to line 16 on page 3. If you are not claiming electronic copies, skip to line 17 on page 3.

PS Form 3526, July 2014 (Page 2 of 4)				
16. Electronic Copy Circulation			Average No. Copies Each Issue During Preceding 12 Months	No. Copies of Single Issue Published Nearest to Filing Date
a. Paid Electronic Copies		▶		
b. Total Paid Print Copies (Line 15c) + Paid Electronic Copies (Line 16a)		▶		
c. Total Print Distribution (Line 15f) + Paid Electronic Copies (Line 16a)		▶		
d. Percent Paid (Both Print & Electronic Copies) (16b divided by 16c × 100)		▶		

☒ I certify that 50% of all my distributed copies (electronic and print) are paid above a nominal price.

17. Publication of Statement of Ownership
☒ If the publication is a general publication, publication of this statement is required. Will be printed
in the   OCTOBER 2022   issue of this publication.   ☐ Publication not required.

18. Signature and Title of Editor, Publisher, Business Manager, or Owner

Malathi Samayan   Date 9/18/2022

Malathi Samayan - Distribution Controller

I certify that all information furnished on this form is true and complete. I understand that anyone who furnishes false or misleading information on this form or who omits material or information requested on the form may be subject to criminal sanctions (including fines and imprisonment) and/or civil sanctions (including civil penalties).

PS Form 3526, July 2014 (Page 3 of 4)   PRIVACY NOTICE: See our privacy policy on www.usps.com

Moving?

Make sure your subscription moves with you!

To notify us of your new address, find your **Clinics Account Number** (located on your mailing label above your name), and contact customer service at:

Email: journalscustomerservice-usa@elsevier.com

800-654-2452 (subscribers in the U.S. & Canada)
314-447-8871 (subscribers outside of the U.S. & Canada)

Fax number: 314-447-8029

Elsevier Health Sciences Division
Subscription Customer Service
3251 Riverport Lane
Maryland Heights, MO 63043

*To ensure uninterrupted delivery of your subscription, please notify us at least 4 weeks in advance of move.